Nesrine Souayeh
Mariem Nouira
Mohamed Frikha

Lumbo-aortic curage in pelvic gynaecological cancers

Nesrine Souayeh
Mariem Nouira
Mohamed Frikha

Lumbo-aortic curage in pelvic gynaecological cancers

interests and controversies

ScienciaScripts

Imprint

Any brand names and product names mentioned in this book are subject to trademark, brand or patent protection and are trademarks or registered trademarks of their respective holders. The use of brand names, product names, common names, trade names, product descriptions etc. even without a particular marking in this work is in no way to be construed to mean that such names may be regarded as unrestricted in respect of trademark and brand protection legislation and could thus be used by anyone.

Cover image: www.ingimage.com

This book is a translation from the original published under ISBN 978-620-6-72295-3.

Publisher:
Sciencia Scripts
is a trademark of
Dodo Books Indian Ocean Ltd. and OmniScriptum S.R.L publishing group

120 High Road, East Finchley, London, N2 9ED, United Kingdom
Str. Armeneasca 28/1, office 1, Chisinau MD-2012, Republic of Moldova, Europe
Printed at: see last page
ISBN: 978-620-8-35667-5

Contents

1 INTRODUCTION

Lymph node involvement, particularly in the lumbo-aortic region, is a major prognostic factor in terms of survival and an essential parameter in the therapeutic strategy for pelvic gynaecological cancers, namely ovarian, endometrial and cervical cancer [1]. The 5-year survival rate falls from 90% to 40% in the case of lymph node involvement for ovarian cancer and from 90% to 30% for endometrial cancer.

There are many indications for lumbo-aortic curage (LAC), and these differ from one gynaecological cancer to another. This surgery may be indicated either as part of systematic staging, or in the presence of major risk factors for lymph node involvement, or in the case of macroscopic lumbo-aortic involvement, and finally in the case of proven pelvic lymph node involvement [2]. In order to be validated, the surgical technique for CLA must comply with a standard in its scope, with the minimum possible complications.

Its direct therapeutic value is still controversial, but numerous studies suggest that CLA has therapeutic potential. In fact, this surgery is part of the concept of complete cytoreduction surgery in the hope of achieving better locoregional control with a better chance of survival [2].

Lumbo-aortic lymph node staging makes it possible to extend the target volume of initial or adjuvant radiotherapy fields, more or less associated with chemotherapy, to the lumbo-aortic territory if metastases are documented at this level, particularly in endometrial and cervical cancer [3].

However, the CLA remains a surgical technique that is fairly advanced in gynaecological carcinology practice, requiring several years of training. The technique is not always easy to perform, due to the proximity of the large vessels and the operating difficulties that can lead to a number of per- and post-operative complications, some of which can be fatal.

With this in mind, we carried out this study, collating the cases of patients treated for pelvic gynaecological cancers and for whom CLA was indicated. Through these cases and a review of the literature, we will :

✓ To clarify the indications and limitations of lumbo-aortic curage.

✓ To describe the intra- and post-operative complications of lumbo-aortic curage.

✓ To determine the current role of lumbo-aortic curage in the treatment of gynaecological cancers.

1. PATIENTS

1.1. Type of study

We carried out a single-centre, retrospective, descriptive, analytical and comparative study of 85 patients treated for gynaecological cancer with an indication for lumbo-aortic curage.

1.2. Scope and location of the study

We conducted the present study over a period of 18 years, from January 2004 to December 2021, in the obstetric gynaecology department of the Ben Arous regional hospital. This is a level IIB maternity hospital in the southern suburbs of Tunis, which provides gynaecological, urogynaecological and carcinological surgery.

1.3. Population studied

1.3.1. Inclusion criteria

All patients were included in this study:

✓ Histologically proven ovarian, endometrial or cervical cancer.

✓ Who has been scheduled for lumbo-aortic curage during primary or second-look surgery.

✓ I had the CLA at the obstetric gynecology department of the Ben Arous regional hospital.

1.3.2. Non-inclusion criteria

Patients with pelvic gynaecological cancer were not included in this study:

✓ Who had no indication for lumbo-aortic curage and who had not been included in our work.

✓ Who had had the CLA in another department.

1.3.3. Exclusion criteria

This study did not include :

✓ Patients lost to follow-up.

✓ Unusable files with missing data.

1.3.4. Judging criteria

✓ The primary outcome was the rate of intra- or post-operative complications related to lumbo-aortic curage.

✓ The secondary endpoints were overall survival and relapse rate, whether or not CLA was used.

2. METHODS

2.1. Data collection

A template listing 125 variables was used to collect the data.

These data were collected from :

• Outpatient follow-up files.

- Departmental hospital records.
- Pathology reports.
- Anaesthesia sheets.
- Operating reports.
- Files from the medical oncology and radiotherapy departments of the Saleh Azaiz Institute in Tunis and Ariana.

2.2. Variables studied

2.2.1. Socio-epidemiological data

We collected the following clinical data for each patient on a standardised form:
- Patient identification (name, age, file number, address, telephone number, etc.).
- Personal and family history
- Menarche and menopause dates
- Gestite and parite
- Notion of infertility
- Contraception and contraceptive methods
- Smoking

2.2.2. Positive diagnosis

2.2.2.1. History and clinical examination

The history clarified the functional signs, the time between the first symptom and the first consultation, and the time between the first consultation and the positive diagnosis.

The clinical examination revealed :
- Assess the patient's general condition and calculate the ASA (American Society of Anaesthesiologists) score (Appendix 1).
- Calculate your body mass index.
- Carry out a gynaecological examination to look for metrorrhagia and cervical or adnexal masses.
- Look for adenopathy.
- Look for clinical signs of distant involvement.
- Classify the tumour according to its clinical stage using the FIGO classification (Appendices 2, 3, 4, 5, 6, 7 and 8).

2.2.2.2. Histology

Confirmation of the diagnosis was obtained either by biopsy (during diagnostic hysteroscopy for endometrial cancer, cervical biopsy for cervical cancer or diagnostic celioscopy in the case of a suspected adnexal mass), or by examination on the operating table.

The histological type was defined according to the WHO classification

(Appendices 9, 10 and 11).

2.2.3. *Assessment of locoregional and distant extension*

All patients in our series underwent thoracic-abdominal-pelvic (TAP) computed tomography (CT) and abdominal-pelvic magnetic resonance imaging (MRI) (Figure 1).

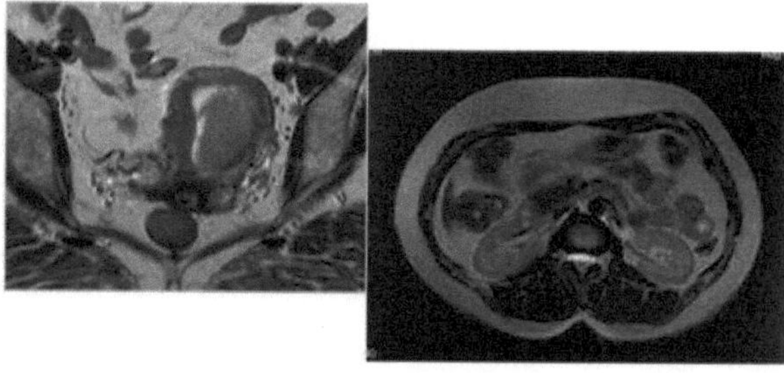

Study of the pelvic and lumbo-aortic gg chains
Small 5mm left exteme iliac
lymph node
No pelvic or lumbo-aortic ADP

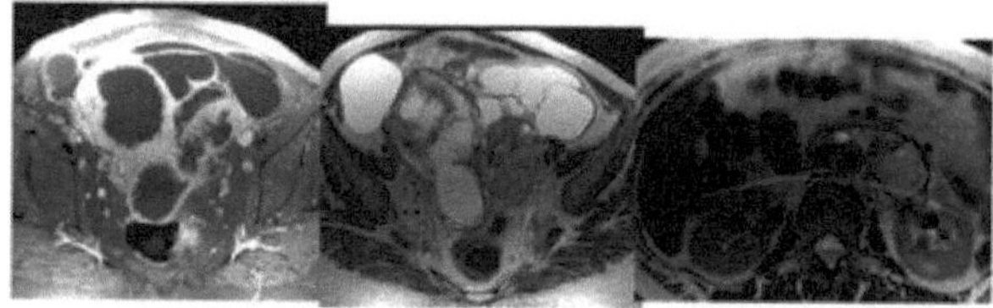

Uterine ADK, ovarian extension; pelvic carcinosis and large latero-aortic metastatic ADP left (same tumour signal as hyper T2 heterogeneous)

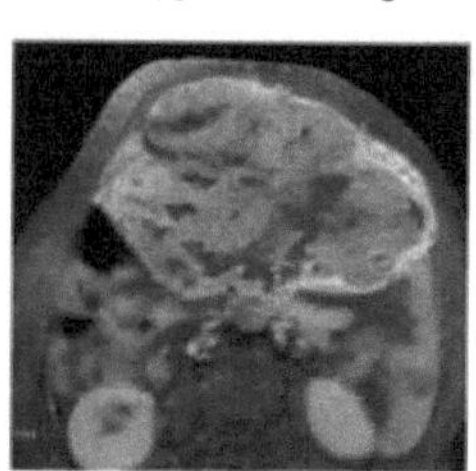

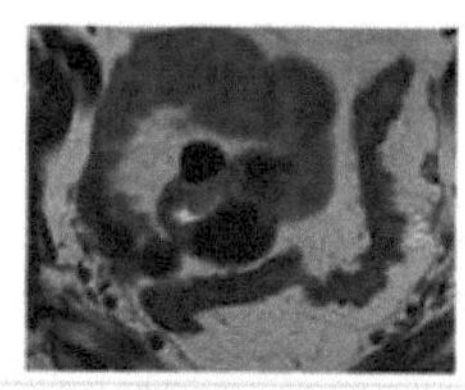

Stage IA clear cell carcinoma(*) Productive right external iliac curage with adenomalacia, all histologically negative

<u>Figure 1:</u> *Assessment of locoregional and distant extension*

2.2.4.   Intraoperative complications

The intraoperative complications reported in our study were necessarily related to lumbo-aortic curage and were classified into five grades according to the new classification of intraoperative complications (**ClassIntra**) published in the British Medical Journal BMJ in August 2020 [4] (Appendix 12).

> **Grade 1** included any deviation from the ideal surgical course without the need for further treatment or intervention: patients with no or few symptoms. Example:

- Above-average bleeding from a small-calibre vessel: self-limiting or definitively controllable with no treatment other than routine coagulation.
- Minimal lesion of the intestinal serosa requiring no further treatment.
- Cauterisation: small skin burn where no treatment is necessary - Rhythm disorder: rhythm disorder (e.g. extrasystoles) with no repercussions.
- **Grade 2** included any deviation from the ideal intraoperative course requiring additional minor treatment or intervention: patient with moderate, non-life-threatening symptoms and no permanent disability. Example:
- Bleeding from a medium-calibre artery or vein: ligation and/or use of Tranexamic acid.
- Non-transmural intestinal lesion requiring one or more sutures.
- Cauterisation: Moderate burn requiring non-invasive wound care.
- Rhythm disorder requiring the administration of an anti-arrhythmic drug without hemodynamic repercussions.

> **Grade 3** included any deviation from the ideal intraoperative course requiring additional moderate treatment or intervention: patients with severe, potentially life-threatening and/or permanently disabling symptoms. Example:

- Bleeding from a large-calibre artery or vein with transient hemodynamic instability: ligation or suture and/or blood transfusion.
- Transmural intestinal lesion requiring segmental resection.
- Cauterisation: Serious burn requiring surgical debridement
- Rhythm disorder requiring the administration of an anti-arrhythmic drug, with transient hemodynamic repercussions.

> **Grade 4** included any deviation from the ideal intraoperative course with the need for urgent major additional treatment or intervention: patient with life-threatening and/or permanently disabling symptoms. Example:

- Life-threatening haemorrhage with splenectomy; massive blood transfusion, stay in intensive care.

- Lesion of a central artery or vein requiring extensive bowel resection.
- Cauterisation: Life-threatening cautery burn requiring intensive care treatment.
- Rhythm disorder requiring electroconversion, defibrillation or admission to a cardiac intensive care unit (CICU).

> **Grade 5**: Intraoperative death of the patient.

2.2.5. *Post-operative complications*

Short- and medium-term postoperative complications were noted either during readmission or as part of the patient's usual follow-up visits. They were described with reference to the Clavien Dindo classification used for postoperative complications (Appendix 13).

2.2.6. *Adjuvant treatment*

The indications for chemotherapy, radiotherapy or curative curietherapy were discussed at the multidisciplinary consultation meeting with the medical oncology and radiotherapy departments of the Abderahmen Mami Hospital in Ariana and the Salah Azaiz Institute, with reference to current recommendations.

2.2.7. *Follow-up*

Monitoring was alternated between gynaecologists, medical oncologists and radiotherapists at a rate of one consultation every 6 months.

Follow-up was carried out by telephone contact with patients or their families until March 2022, and by consulting patients' files when they completed their treatment at either the Abderrahmen Mami Ariana Hospital or the Salah Azaiz Institute.

The prognostic data collected were :

✓ Overall survival (OS): defined as the time in months between the date of diagnosis and the date of death or last news.

✓ Recurrence (or relapse): defined as locoregional recurrence of the disease or distant metastasis after curative carcinological treatment.

✓ Recurrence-free survival (RFS): defined as the time in months between the date of diagnosis and the date of occurrence of an event. Events included in the RFS were relapses and death from any cause.

We have calculated the SG at 1, 2 and 3 years as well as the SSR at 3 years.

2.3. Operating technique for lumbo-aortic curage

The technique adopted by our team is that described in 1998 by Querleu [5]. The open CLA technique has not undergone any major changes or progress, since the laparoscopic and, more recently, the robotic approach have taken over and are currently the most widely used techniques in the world. The lack of an adequate technical platform for these surgical innovations makes recourse to the laparotomy route inevitable in the case of the patients in our study.

Ж *Description of the technique* [5]:

Cellulo-ganglion sampling is systematic: latero-aortic, right and left common iliac, pre-aortic-caval, and latero-caval.

The principle of lymphadenectomy is based on strict dissection in the plane of the adventitia of the main vessels and the interface planes of the various adipose structures (peri-renal fat, mesenteric fat). The aim was to identify the lymph node slits and perform selective hemostasis and lymphostasis.

For para-aortic and common iliac lymphadenectomy, three fundamental landmarks (the psoas muscle, the left ureter and the common iliac artery) are highlighted with any dissection. The left lateral border of the aorta is followed to access the left renal vein. From the anterior surface of the aorta arise the inferior mesenteric artery, which is respected, and the left ovarian artery, which is coagulated and sectioned, allowing access to the pre-aortic lymph nodes. The nodes medial to the common iliac artery are then removed after identification of the promontory and left common iliac vein. The laterocaval, retrovascular and right common iliac lymph nodes are then removed by detaching between the promontory and the mesosigmoid and progressing tangentially to the origin of the left common iliac vein and the bifurcation of the vena cava. The laterocaval lymph nodes can be accessed either anteriorly to the aorta, or more rarely by detaching the aorta and then the vena cava from the spine (Figures 2 and 3).

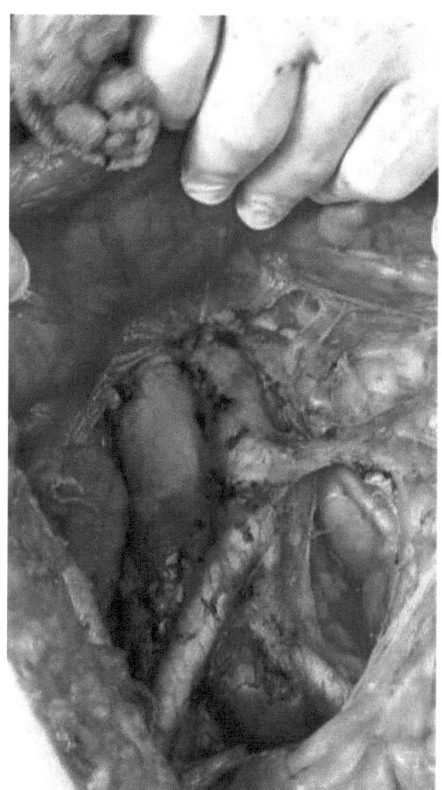

**Figure 2:** *CLA for stage II ovarian adenocarcinoma*

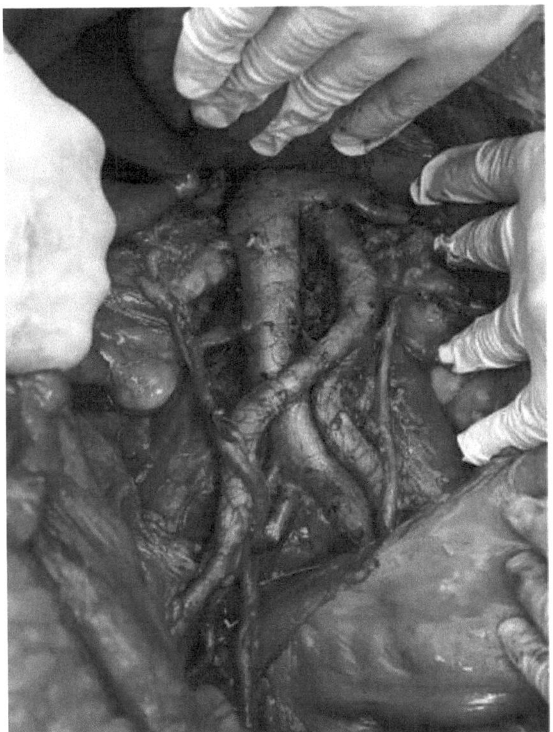

Figure 3: CLA for endometroid carcinoma stage Ib grade 3

2.4. Statistical methods

Data entry and statistical analysis were carried out using SPSS 26.0fr software.

2.4.1. Descriptive analysis

We carried out a descriptive study of patients with pelvic gynaecological cancer requiring lumbo-aortic curage. Qualitative variables were described according to their percentage distribution with 95% confidence intervals (95% CI). For quantitative variables, the analysis was based on the presentation of means and standard deviations when the distribution was normal and, in the opposite case, on the median with the interquartile range.

The normality of the distribution was checked using the Kolmogorov-Smirnov and Shapiro Wilk tests.

2.4.2. Statistical tests

We divided our population into two groups:

✓ Group with CLA. : CLA

✓ Group that did not take the CLA: without CLA

Data from patients in the two groups were compared. For quantitative variables, we used Student's t test, and the results were presented with their p significance levels. For qualitative variables, we used Pearson's chi-square test. The results were presented with their p, relative risks (RR) and 95% CI. Non-parametric tests were used whenever necessary.

The results were presented in the form of tables and graphs.

Overall survival and relapse curves were calculated using the Kaplan-Meier method.

A multivariate analysis using top-down logistic regression (Wald) was performed by introducing all factors with p values < 0.05. Each factor identified was then presented with its adjusted relative risk and 95% CI.

In all tests, the p threshold was set at 5% $(p< 0.05)$ and the multivariate analysis was performed using SPSS 26.0 Fr software.

2.5. Bibliographic research

A bibliographical search was carried out by consulting the digital data available on PubMed, Cochrane library, Google Scholar, etc. Theses available in Tunisian faculties of medicine as well as foreign doctoral theses in medicine using the key words: lumbo-aortic curage, pelvic gynecological cancer, limits and intra- and post-operative complications, morbidity, mortality, recurrence and survival.

The references have been ordered according to the Vancouver model.

2.6. Ethical considerations and conflicts of interest

We declare that we have no conflict of interest in this work and that we have respected medical ethics in all the cases that have been treated. No patient was paid and no funding was provided by a pharmaceutical industry.

Given the retrospective nature of the study, no consent could be obtained from the patients included in this study regarding the use of the personal data mentioned on the medical records.

Strict anonymity of individual data was maintained throughout the study. Only the principal investigator knew the identity of the patients.

The agreement of the ethics committee was not obtained for this study, given its retrospective nature.

1. DESCRIPTIVE STUDY

1.1. Study population

Of 85 patients managed for gynaecological cancer in our study with an indication for lumbo-aortic curage, 30 were excluded. A total of 55 cases were included in our study (Figure 4).

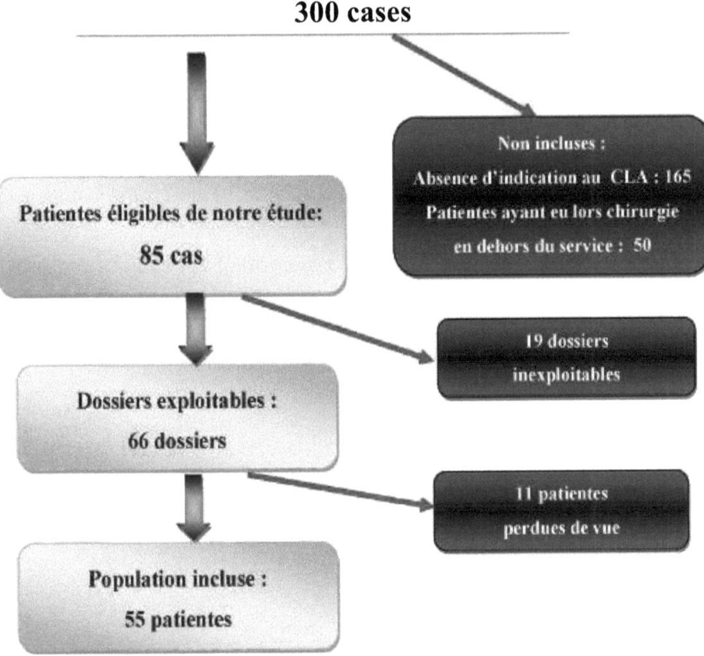

Figure 4: Flow Chart for patient inclusion

1.2. Epidemiological data

1.2.1. Breakdown by type of cancer

Figure 5 shows the distribution of patients in our study according to the type of gynaecological cancer.

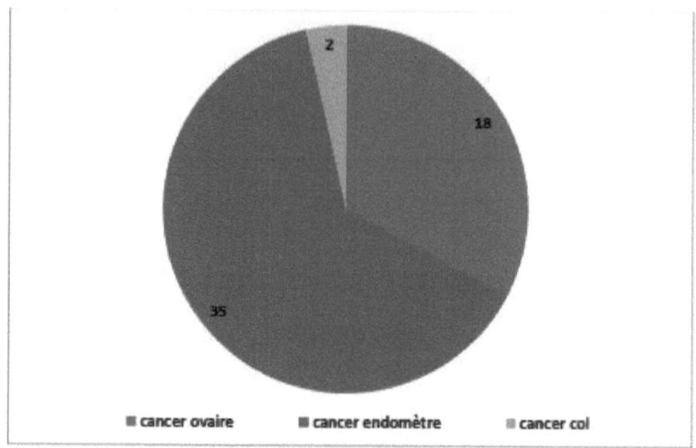

Figure 5 : Distribution of patients by type of cancer

1.1.2. Age

The mean age of the patients in our study was 58.4 years (± 8.4), with extremes of 39 and 75 years.

The majority of patients (52.7%) were aged over 60 at the time of diagnosis (Figure 6).

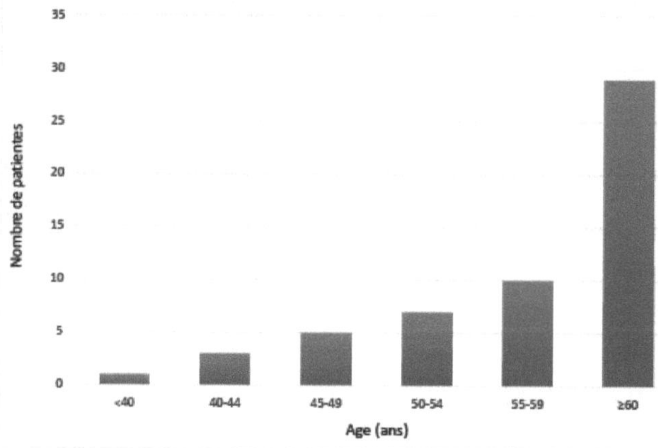

Figure 6: Age distribution of patients

1.1.3. Family history of cancer

Eleven patients had a history of gynaecological cancer, i.e. 20% of our population (Figure 7).

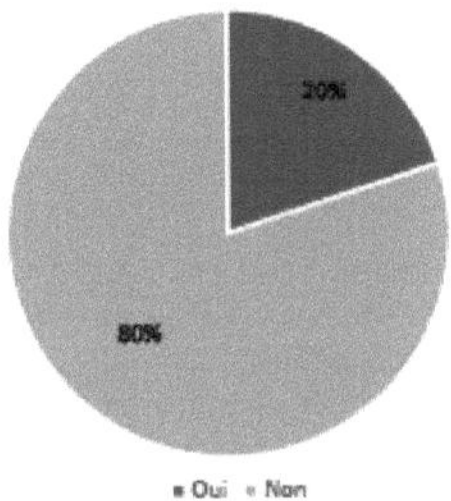

__Figure 7:__ Breakdown of patients by gynaecological history

1.1.4. *Medical history*

Arterial hypertension and diabetes were present in 47% and 42% of patients respectively.

Other comorbidities noted in this series were dyslipidemia and coronary insufficiency (6 cases), associated breast cancer (2 cases), anemia (1 case) and associated ovarian cyst (1 case) (Figure 8).

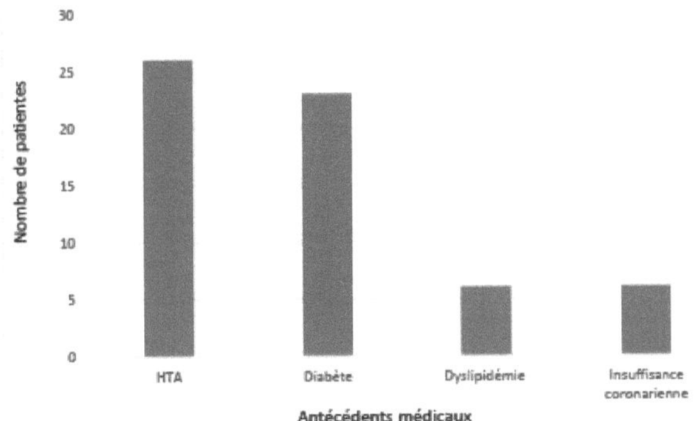

__Figure 8:__ Breakdown of patients by medical history

1.1.5. *Previous surgery*

Abdominal scarring was noted in 17 patients (25.5%).

The surgical antecedents observed in the patients in our study are summarised in Figure 9.

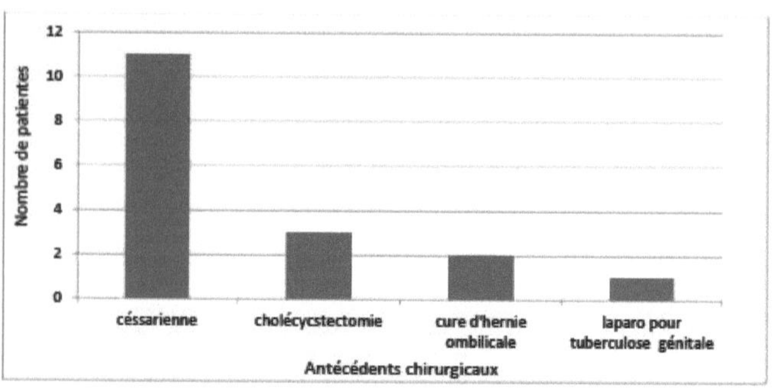

<u>Figure 9:</u> Breakdown by surgical antecedents

1.1.6.   Body mass index (BMI)

The average body mass index was 32.7 kg.m^2 (± 5.97) with a minimum of 20 and a maximum of 45.9 kg.m2.

Overweight was noted in 17 patients (30.9%), while obesity was confirmed in 34 patients (61.8% of the series) (Figure 10).

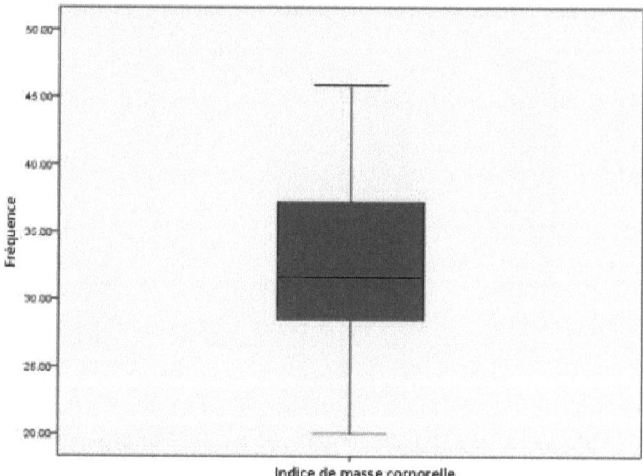

<u>Figure 10:</u> Breakdown by body mass index

1.1.7. Gynecological history

1.1.7.1.   Menarche

Three cases of precocious puberty were noted, with a median of 12 years and extremes between 9 and 16 years.

1.1.7.2.   Gestite / Parite

The median gestational age and parity was 3, with extremes of 0 and 13. Nulliparity was noted in 30.9% of patients (17 cases).

1.1.7.3.   Hormonal contraception

Hormonal contraception was used in 6 of our patients (28.6%).

1.1.7.4.   Menopause

16

The majority of patients (81.8%) were menopausal. Late menopause was found in 35% of cases (Figure 11).

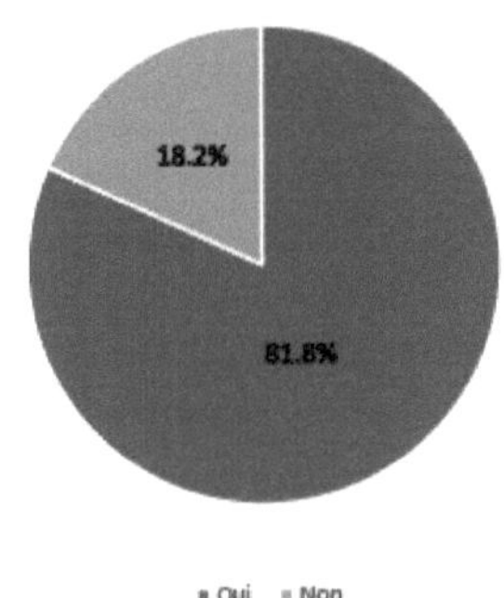

__Figure 11:__ Breakdown of patients by menopause

1.1.8.   *ASA score*

Patients were distributed according to ASA score as follows (Figure 12)

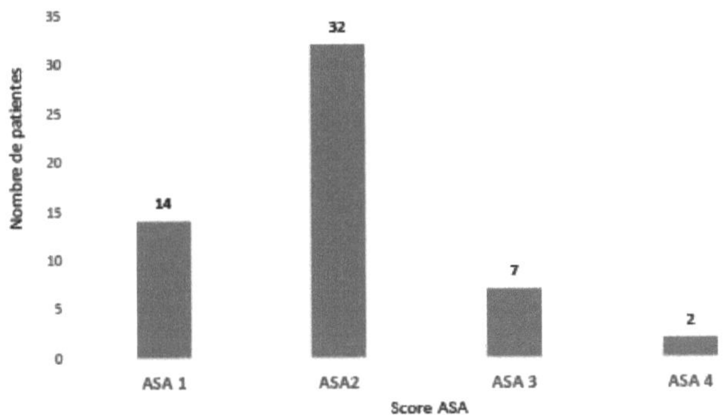

__Figure 12:__ Distribution of patients according to ASA score

1.3. Symptomatology

1.3.1.   *Circumstances of discovery*

Metrorrhagia and the discovery of a pelvic mass were the most common symptoms in our series, accounting for 45.5% of cases. Figure 13 summarises the different signs that prompted patients to consult a doctor.

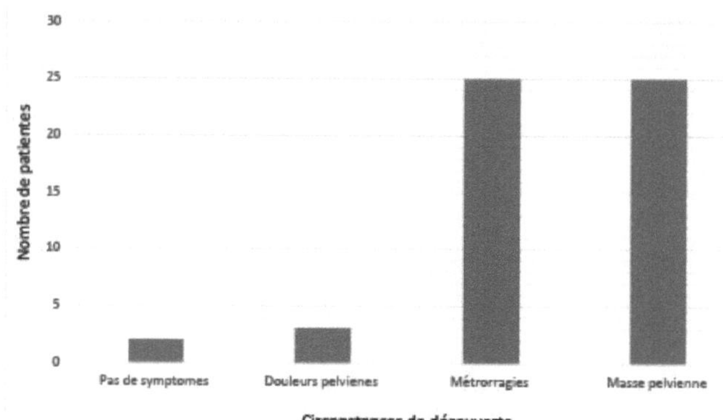

__Figure 13:__ Breakdown of patients by reason for discovery

1.3.2.   *Time between symptoms and consultation*

The average time between the onset of symptoms and the first consultation was 2 months (+/- 0.95), ranging from 0 to 60 months. One patient, aged 62 at the time she was treated, complained of pelvic pain which she ignored. She consulted after 5 years and was found to have endometrial cancer. In addition, two patients had consulted for post-menopausal metrorrhagia within 07 and 15 years respectively.

1.3.3.   *Delay between symptomatology and diagnosis*

The mean time from onset of symptoms to positive diagnosis was 4 months ($\pm$ 0.95), with extremes of between 1 and 61 months.

1.4. Diagnostic procedures

1.4.1.   *Clinical data*

Abdominal examination revealed an abdominal mass in 3 cases in our series, all related to ovarian cancer. Percussion led us to suspect peritoneal ascites in 4 cases of ovarian cancer.

Speculum examination and vaginal touch combined with abdominal palpation enabled us to detect three suspicious cervical masses, two of which were subsequently related to cervical cancer and only one to endometrial cancer that had invaded the cervix.

1.4.2.   *Imaging data*

Diagnostic orientation was based on endovaginal ultrasound, which was performed in all patients in our series.

Only 7 patients did not undergo abdominopelvic MRI, all of whom were managed before 2009.

6 other patients did not undergo a TAP scan as part of the extension work-up.

1.4.3.   *Tumour markers*

CA 125 was requested in 16 patients with a suspected ovarian cyst, i.e. in 80%

of cases (16/20). Its value was pathological in 87.5% of cases (14/16).

1.4.4. *Hysteroscopy / Diagnostic laparoscopy*

Hysteroscopy was performed in all cases of endometrial cancer and in two cases of ovarian cancer, in response to the occurrence of metrorrhagia.

All patients with suspected ovarian cancer underwent primary diagnostic fluoroscopy to perform intraoperative staging and to confirm radiological findings.

All patients had undergone additional biopsies (endometrium/ovary) following these two endoscopic procedures.

Three patients had undergone cervical biopsy under anaesthetic in the operating theatre, resulting in two cervical cancers and one patient with extension of endometrial cancer to the cervix.

1.4.5. *Anatomopathology*

An extemporaneous examination was performed in 9 patients when there was a discrepancy between the radiology and the intraoperative appearance. All these patients had ovarian cancer.

1.4.5.1. Ovarian cancer

Out of 18 cases of ovarian cancer:	16	(88.9%) were of the type serous adenocarcinoma (90%), and two of endometroid type. Thirteen patients (72, 2%) had FIGO stage III classification.

Two patients had FIGO stage 1. They had synchronous endometrial cancer.

1.4.5.2. Endometrial cancer

Endometrial cancer was endometroid in 71.4% of cases (25/35) and non-endometroid in the remaining 28.6%.

Twenty-seven cases of endometrial cancer (77.1%) were diagnosed at stage 1 of the FIGO classifications, including 16 cases at stage IC of the old FIGO 1989 classification.

1.4.5.3. Cervical cancer

Our series included 2 cases of squamous cell carcinoma of the cervix diagnosed at FIGO 2018 stage IB1.

1.4.5.4. Presence of lymphatic emboli

The presence of lymphatic emboli on anatomopathological examination was noted in 9% of cases, i.e. 5 patients in our study. Two had cervical cancer and 3 had endometrial cancer (Table I).

Table I: Classification of cases in the study population

Classification FIGO	Cervical cancer	Cancer of The endometrium	Ovarian cancer
2002-2009 FIGO 1989	-	21 cases -IC stage: **16**	8 cases -Stage II: **2**

				-Stage II: **2** -Stage III: **3**	-Stage III: **6**
2010-2018	FIGO2009	- -- - -		**8 cases** Stage I(*): **2** Stage I A type 2: **1** IB stage: **3** Stage II: **2**	**8 cases** -Stage I(*): **2** -Stage IIB: **1** -Stage IIIB: **2** -Stage IIIC: **3**
2019-2021	FIGO 2018	**2 cases** (stage IB1) - - -		**6 cases** Stage I, type 2: **2** IB stage: **3** Stage II: **1**	**2 cases** - Stage III B: **1** - stage IIIC: **1**
Total cases		**2**		**35**	**18**

(*) Case of synchronous ovarian and uterine cancer.

1.5. Treatment: lymph node dissection

1.5.1. Pelvic curage

Pelvic curage was performed in all patients in our series.

1.5.2. Lumbo-aortic curage

Three quarters of our patients benefited from a complete pelvic and lumbo-aortic curage, while the remaining 25.5% (14 patients) underwent only a single pelvic curage, even though the MLC was indicated.

A total of 41 patients underwent pelvic and lumbo-aortic curage: 23 had endometrial cancer, 17 ovarian cancer and one cervical cancer (Figure 14).

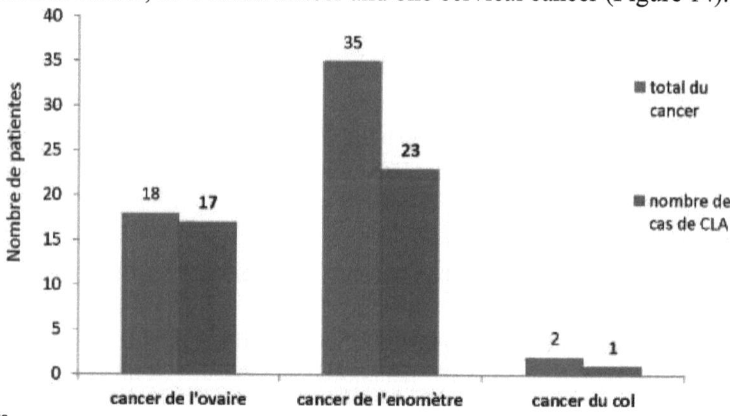

Figure 14: Distribution of lumbo-aortic curage according to cancers

1.5.3. Number of lymph nodes collected

The median number of nodes removed during curage was 28 per curage, with extremes ranging from 10 to 58 nodes.

The median number of lumbo-aortic lymph nodes removed was 8, with extremes of between 2 and 19 nodes.

For cases of ovarian cancer, a positive CLA was noted in 10 patients out of 17 practical CLAs (58%) and all were advanced stage (IIB and above). In all these cases, pelvic curage was also positive. In addition, two patients (11%) had pelvic lymph node involvement without associated lumbo-aortic invasion.

For endometrial cancer, a positive CLA was noted in 6 patients (26%). In a third of cases, the cancer was early stage and located in the uterus (Table II).

Table II: Breakdown of cases by type and stage of cancer

Type of Cancer	Number of cases	CLA done	CLA positive	Stadium
Ovary	18	17	10	9: stage III 1: stage IIB
Endometrium	35	23	6	2: IB stage 1: stage II 3: stage III
Collar	2	1	0	

CLA: lumbo-aortic curage

1.5.4.   *Time required for cleaning*

The median operating time for the entire surgical procedure, for all cancers combined, was 5 hours (± 0.11), with extremes of between 2 and 8 hours.

The average time required for pelvic and lumbo-aortic curage was 185 minutes plus or minus 15 minutes, with a minimum estimated at 105 minutes and a maximum estimated at 280 minutes.

CLA is associated with a prolongation of operating time of between 1 and 3 hours, with an average prolongation of 1 hour and 10 minutes.

1.5.5.   *Complications of curage*

1.5.5.1.   **Intraoperative complications**

We noted the occurrence of 30 complications during the intraoperative stage. According to the new "ClassIntra" classification of intraoperative events, these complications were distributed according to their grade as follows: Grade 1: 50%, Grade 2: 26.7%, Grade 3: 20% and Grade 4: 3.3% (Figure 15).

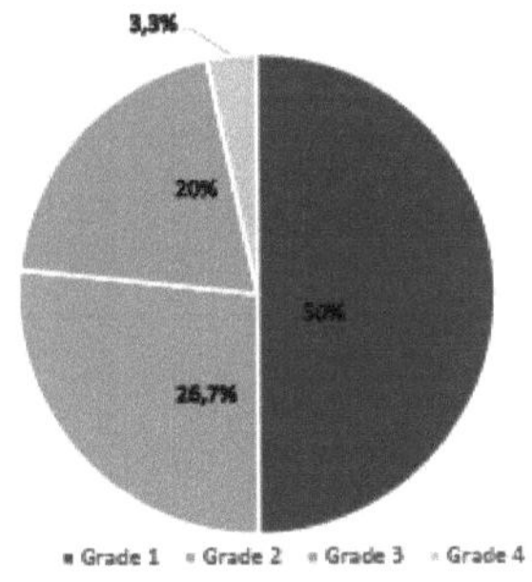

Figure 15: Breakdown of intraoperative complications by grade

✓ Most of the Grade 1 complications (98.2%) were minor bleeding. In addition, there was one case of benign arrhythmia such as ventricular extrasystole with no clinical repercussions and spontaneous regression.

✓ Grade 2 complications included one case of non-transmural digestive lesion requiring suture and 7 cases of vascular bleeding from a medium-calibre vessel that was ligated in time.

✓ Grade 3 complications included 6 cases of large-calibre vascular lesions with hemodynamic instability requiring vascular ligation or suture.

✓ Only one grade 4 complication was noted, involving life-threatening haemorrhage requiring massive transfusion (Table III).

✓ No cases of death (grade 5) were reported.

Table III: Breakdown of intraoperative complications by grade

Grade of intraoperative complication according to ClassIntra	Number of cases	Type
Grade 1 :	15	Bleeding: 14 Digestive lesion: 0 Burns: 0 Arrhythmia: 1
Grade 2 :	8	Bleeding: 7 Digestive lesion: 1 Burns: 0 Arrhythmia: 0
Grade 3 :	6	Bleeding: 6 Digestive lesion: 0 Burns: 0 Arrhythmia: 0
Grade 4 :	1	Bleeding: 1 Digestive lesion: 0 Burn: 0 Arrhythmia: 0

1.5.5.2. Post-operative complications

We noted 43 postoperative complications. According to the "Clavien-Dindo" classification of postoperative events, these

Complications are broken down by grade as follows (Figure 16):

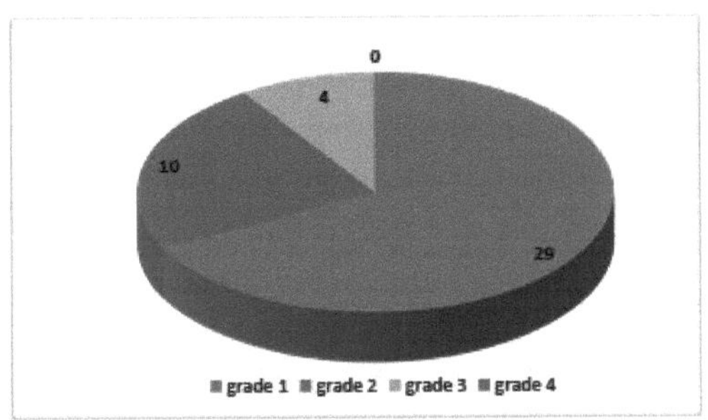

Figure 16: Breakdown of post-operative complications by grade

> Grade 1 complications: we noted 14 cases of postoperative fever, 7 cases of wall abscess and 8 cases of prolonged ileus of functional origin.

> Grade 2 complications: We noted the occurrence of thromboembolic complications in 4 patients. In addition, 6 patients required a blood transfusion postoperatively.

> For Grade 3 complications: 4 patients required repeat surgery. Two were carcinological, due to local recurrence of cervical cancer operable on the vaginal slice, and one was endometrial cancer. These two patients were in the no CLA group. The other two cases of revision surgery were for eventration on median laparotomy (Table IV).

Table IV: Breakdown of post-operative complications by grade

Grade of post-operative complication according to the Clavien-Dindo method	Number of cases	Type
Grade 1	29	Fever: 14 Wall thickness: 7 Ildus extends contract: 8
Grade 2	10	Complication TE: 4 Transfusions: 6
Grade 3	4	Surgical revision: 4
Grade 4	0	

1.5.5.3. Operative morbidity

The average length of hospital stay was 28 days, with a minimum of 14 and a maximum of 60 days.

In addition, only one patient required transfer to an intensive care unit; this was the patient who presented the only grade 4 intraoperative complication (hemodynamic instability).

1.5.5.4. Specific complications of curage

These complications were lymphoedemas of the lower limbs in 6 cases (10.9%) and lymphoceles in 11 cases (20%).

1.6. Study of overall survival

Regardless of the type of cancer, the median overall survival for our population was 38 months, with extremes of 5 and 144 months.

The median overall survival for endometrial cancer in our series was 36 months [12-98 months] while that for ovarian cancer was 48 months [5-87 months] (Figure 17).

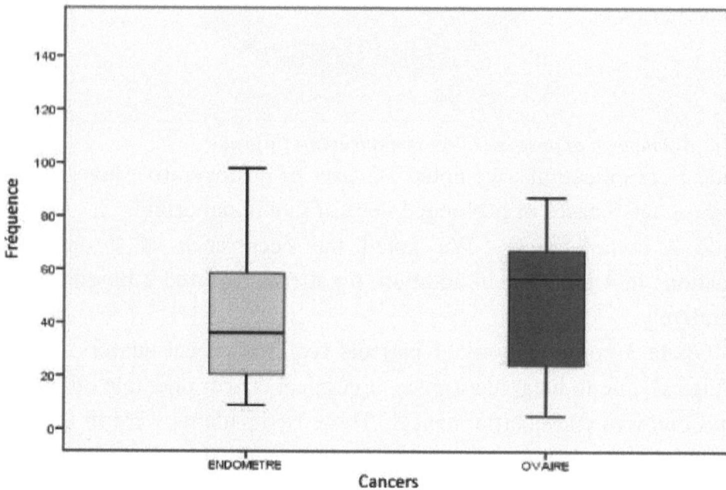

Figure 17: Overall survival by cancer

1.6.1.   *Survival to 1 year*

The 1-year survival rate for all cancers combined was 92.7%. In our series, two cases of ovarian cancer (3.8%) and one case of endometrial cancer (1.9%) did not survive beyond one year. They both belonged to the CLA group (Figure 18).

1.6.2.   *Survival 2 years*

Two-year survival for all cancers combined was 67.3%. For endometrial and ovarian cancer, it was 62.8% and 77.7% respectively (Figure 18).

1.6.3.   *Survival 3 years*

The 3-year survival rate for all cancers combined in our series was 56.4%. For endometrial cancer it was 51.4% and 66.6% for ovarian cancer (Figure 18).

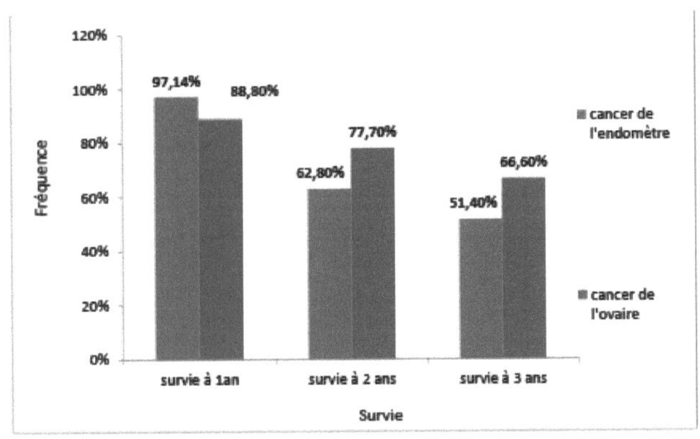

Figure 18: Survival at 1, 2 and 3 years by type of cancer

1.7. Study of recidivism

We recorded 7 cases (12.7%) of recurrence in our series; 3 for endometrial cancer, 3 for ovarian cancer and one case of cervical cancer. The 3 cases of recurrence of ovarian cancer were all at an advanced stage (IIB and III). For endometrial cancer, recurrence was noted at different stages of the cancer. The mean time to recurrence was 26.14 months. This **was** 23.3 months for ovarian cancer and 18.3 months for endometrial cancer (Table V).

Table V: Study of recidivism

Recidivism	Age	type of cance	FIGO cancer r stage	CLA does	Time to recidivism (months)
1er cases	52	Ovary	IIB	+	18
2eme cases	41	Ovary	IIIC	+	45
3eme cases	60	Ovary	IIIC	+	7
4eme cases	58	Endometrium	IB	-	12
5eme cases	52	Endometrium	III	+	6
6eme cases	49	Endometrium	III	-	37
7eme cases	55	collar	IB1	-	17

2. DATA ANALYSIS

2.1. Factors associated with non-repair of lumbo-aortic curage

2.1.1. Age

The mean age for the "without lumbo-aortic curing" group was 60.85 years, compared with 57.56 years for the "with LA curing" group.

There was no significant difference in age between the two groups.

2.1.2. Body mass index

The median body mass index was 37.2 kg/.m² for the group without curing and

30.4 for the group with curing.

There was a significant difference in body mass index between the two groups (p = 0.02) with an area under the curve equal to 0.77 and a threshold value of 34. Thus, above a body mass index value of 34, the risk of failure of lumbo-aortic curage was greater (Figure 19).

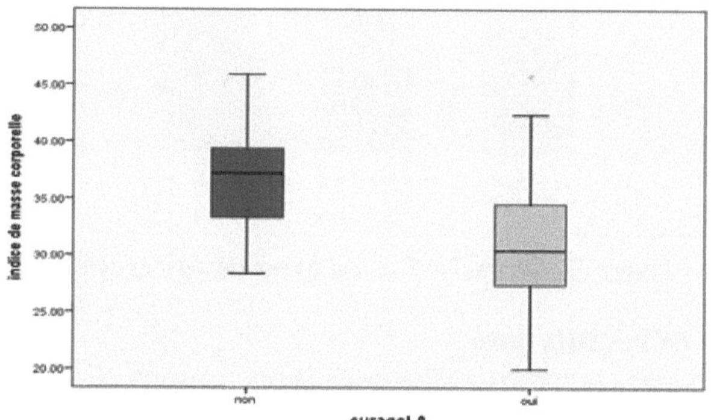

***Figure 19:** CLA realisation as a function of body mass index*

Of the patients who had not undergone lumbo-aortic curage, 85.7% were obese, whereas 53.7% of the patients who had undergone LAC were obese. The difference between the two groups was statistically significant (p=0.03) with a relative risk of 0.193 [0.38-0.97]).

2.1.3. *ASA score*

Regarding the ASA score, the median in the two groups was comparable (median equal to 2) and there was no difference between the two groups (p=0.43).

2.1.4. *Abdominal scar*

Of the patients who had not had CLA, 5 had a scarred abdomen (35.7%) compared with 8 in the CLA group (19.5%). The difference between the two groups was not statistically significant (p=0.3).

In addition, 3 of the patients who had not received CLA (21.4%) had adhesions discovered intraoperatively, compared with 13 in the CLA group (31.7%). The "intraoperative adhesions" parameter was not as significant (p=0.465).

2.1.5. *Complications of pelvic curage*

In our study, 65% of the patients (9 cases) in the group without CLA had had a per-operative complication during pelvic curage which meant that CLA was not performed. Conversely, in the CLA group, 7.3% of patients (3 cases) completed their lumbo-aortic curage despite the occurrence of a complication during pelvic curage.

The difference between these two groups was significant (p=0.002) with a relative risk of 0.105 [0.022-0.512] (Figure 20).

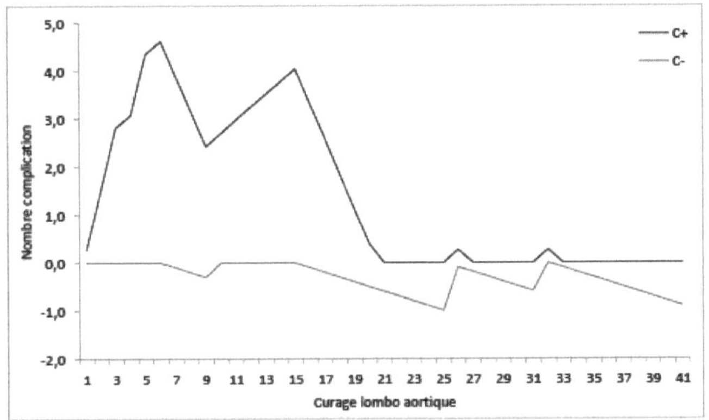

Figure 20: CLA as a function of the number of complications during pelvic curettage

2.1.6. Operator experience

There was a significant difference between the two groups in terms of experience of the surgical team. The median years of experience was 14 years in the CLA group compared with 7 years in the non-CLA group (p = 0.04) (Figure 21).

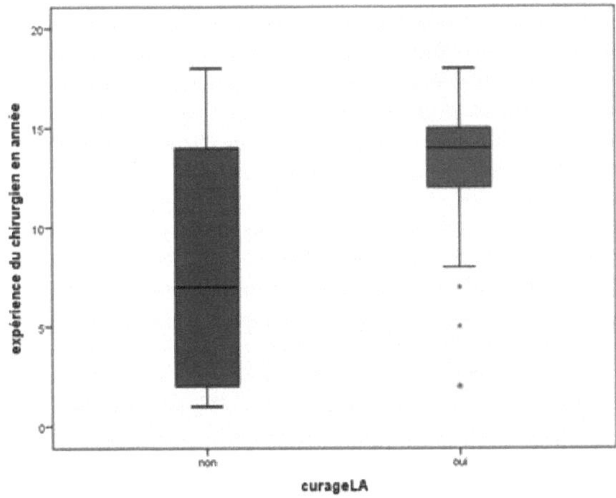

Figure 21: CLA according to surgeon's experience in years

2.1.7. Type of cancer

In the CLA 94.4% group, 17 out of 18 ovarian cancer patients had undergone lumbo-aortic curage, whereas the same procedure was performed in only 65.7% (23 out of 35 cases) of endometrial cancer patients. The difference between the two groups was statistically significant (p=0.05).

In a multivariate study, only the experience of the surgical team (p=0.001) and the presence of complications during pelvic curage (p=0.001) were independent factors in the failure to perform lumbo-aortic curage (Table VI).

<u>*Table VI:*</u> *Multivariate study of factors influencing CLA performance*

	P	*OR (IC95%)*
Type of cancer	**0.184**	**6.259 (0.419 - 93.477)**
Obesite	**0.755**	**1.435 (0.148 - 13.874)**
Complications of pelvic curage	0.001	13.030 (7.732 - 22.554)
Operator experience	0.001	1.411 (1.153 - 1.727)

p: significance level, CI: confidence interval

2.2. Morbidity and complications of lumbo-aortic curage
2.2.1.   Length of stay

The length of hospital stay for patients was comparable for both groups: 31 days on average for the CLA group versus 29 days for the non-CLA group (Figure 22).

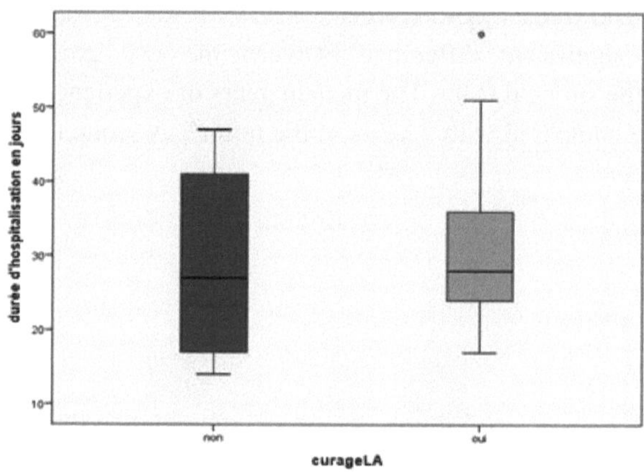

<u>*Figure 22:*</u> *Length of hospital stay according to whether or not CLA was performed*

2.2.2.   Intraoperative complications
✓ .2.2.1. Number of complications

We found a complication rate of around 0.98 on average per operation for the CLA group, compared with 0.21 on average for the group without curage. This difference was statistically significant (p=0.0001).

✓ .2.2.2. Grade of complications

✓ For grade 1 complications:

A total of 10 per-operative complications were noted in the CLA group, compared with 4 in the group without curage. The difference was not statistically significant (p = 0.74).

✓ For grade 2 complications:

For grade 2 complications, we counted 28.6% in the no CLA group and 9.8% in the CLA group. The difference was not significant (p=0.085).

✓ For grade 3 complications:

Three grade 3 complications were noted in each group, with respective percentages of 7.3% and 21.4%, with no significant difference (p=0.144).

✓ For grade 4 complications:

Only one grade 4 complication was noted in our population and this was in the CLA group.

2.2.3. *Post-operative complications*

■ Postoperative fever was present in 14 cases, i.e. in 9 cases (22%) in the CLA group and in 5 cases (35.7%) in the group without curage. The difference was not significant between the two groups (p=0.307).

■ Wall abscess was a postoperative complication in 7 cases in our study; 4 in the CLA group (9.8%) and 3 (21.4%) in the group without curage. The difference between the two groups was not significant (p= 0.258).

■ Thromboembolic complications occurred in 4 cases, all in the CLA group, with no significant difference between the two groups (p=0.225).

■ Lymphoedema of the lower limbs was present postoperatively in 6 patients: 1 (7.1%) in the group without curage and 5 (12.2%) in the CLA group. The difference between the two groups was not significant (p=0.601).

■ A lymphocele was found in 11 cases: 10 (24.4%) in the CLA group and 1 (7.1%) in the group without curage, with no significant difference between the two groups (p=0.164).

■ Prolonged ileus was noted in 8 cases: 7 (17%) in the CLA group compared with 1 case (7%) in the group without curage, with no significant difference between the two groups (p=0.363).

■ Revision surgery was indicated in 11 patients, including 4 (28.6%) in the group without curage and 7 (17.1%) in the CLA group. There was no significant difference between the two groups (Table VII).

Table VII: *Description of intraoperative and postoperative complications according to whether or not CLA was performed*

		CLA Group	Group without cleaning	Value of p
Length of stay (days)		31	29	NS
Complications per operations	Number of intraoperative complications	17	13	0.0008
	Grade 1 complications	24.3%	28.5%	NS
	Grade 2 complications	9.8%	28.6%	NS
	Grade 3 complications	7.3%	21.4%	NS
	Complication grade 4	2.4%	0	NS
Complications per	Post-operative fever	22%	35.7%	NS
	Abces of the wall	9.8%	21.4%	NS
	Thromboembolic	9.8%	0	NS

	complications			
post-operative	Transfusion	12.1%	7.1%	NS
	Lymphoedema	12.2%	7.1%	NS
	Lymphocele	24.4%	7.1%	NS
	Ildus extends contract	17%	7.1%	NS
Surgical revision		17.1%	28.6%	NS

CLA: lumbo-aortic curage, p: degree of significance, NS: not significant

2.3. Recurrence of the disease

We noted the occurrence of tumour recurrence in 7 patients: 5 (35%) in the non-CLA group and 2 (4.87%) in the CLA group. The difference was significant between the two groups (p=0.002).

In our series, irrespective of the type and stage of the cancer, CLA was associated with a lower rate of recurrence.

> For endometrial cancer :

The relative risk of recurrence was 0.13 (0.021- 0.84). The recurrence rate in the non-curage group was 16.6%, whereas it was 4.3% lower in the CLA group, but the difference was not significant (p= 0.21).

The 3 patients who had a recurrence were stage IB (1 patient in the non-CLA group) and stage III for the other two patients (CLA group). Statistical analysis showed that there was a significant difference in favour of CLA in the early stages of endometrial cancer (p=0.0009). However, there was no difference in recurrence between the two groups in the advanced stages (p=0.89).

In our series, CLA was associated with a lower rate of recurrence in early endometrial cancer.

> For ovarian cancer:

The recurrence rate in the CLA group was 21.42%, whereas the patient who did not undergo curage had no recurrence. The difference was not significant (p= 0.64).

All the patients who presented a recurrence had an advanced stage of cancer (3/14) and they had all had a CLA. Comparison between the two groups showed no significant differences (p=0.58).

In our series, the occurrence of recurrence of ovarian cancer was not related to whether or not CLA was performed. Recurrence was more frequent in advanced forms (Table VIII).

Table VIII: Recurrence rates by type of cancer and whether or not CLA was performed

Type of cancer	Recidivism	CLA Group	Group without cleaning	Value of p
Rate of recidivism in the series		4.87%	35%	**0.002** significant
	Recidivism rate	1/23	2/12	0.21
Endometrial cancer	Early stage	0/11	1/11	**0.0009**

				significant
	Advanced stage	1/24	1/24	0.89
Ovarian cancer	Recidivism rate	3/14	0/1	0.64
	Advanced stage	3/10	0/1	0.58

p: degree of significance, CLA: lumbo-aortic curage

2.4. Patient survival

2.4.1. Survival in both groups

Regardless of the type of pelvic gynaecological cancer, overall survival in the CLA group was 45 months compared with 36 months in the non-CLA group, and there was no significant difference between the two groups (Figure 23).

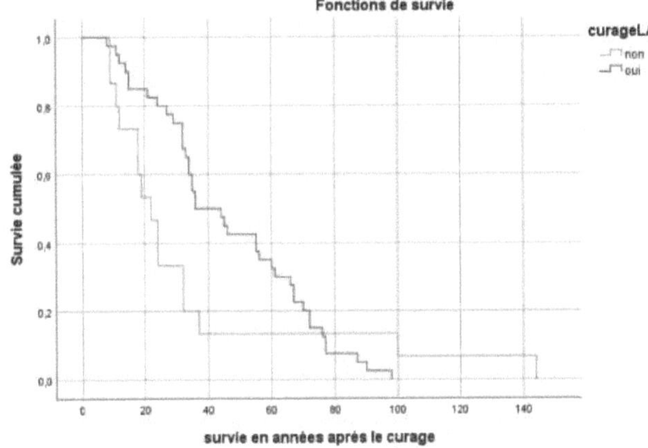

Figure 23: Overall survival curve for the "CLA" and "no CLA" groups

2.4.2. Survival in both groups according to cancer type

We compared the two groups in terms of survival according to the type of cancer.

✓ For endometrial cancer, there was no difference between the two groups in terms of overall survival, 1-year survival, 2-year survival. However, 3-year survival was better in the CLA group with a significant difference (p=0.02).

✓ For ovarian cancer, overall survival was better for the CLA group (46.65 vs 37 months) but the difference was not significant (p=0.68). Similarly, there was no difference between the two groups in terms of survival at 1 year, 2 years and 3 years.

2.4.3. Relapse-free survival

> For endometrial cancer (Figure 24A) :

Recurrence-free survival was better in the CLA group and the difference was statistically significant (p=0.002) at 23 months in the non-CLA group and 38 months in the CLA group.

Recurrence-free survival at 3 years was 61% for the CLA group compared with 16.7% for the group without curage. The difference was significant (p= 0.002) and the RR was 7.77 (1.37- 44).

> For ovarian cancer (Figure 24B) :

Recurrence-free survival was better in the CLA group but the difference was not significant between the two groups, with a rate of 45 vs 37 months.

Recurrence-free survival at 3 years was 57.1% for the CLA group, while the only patient in the non-CLA group survived 3 years without recurrence of the disease.

disease and the difference was not significant (Table IX).

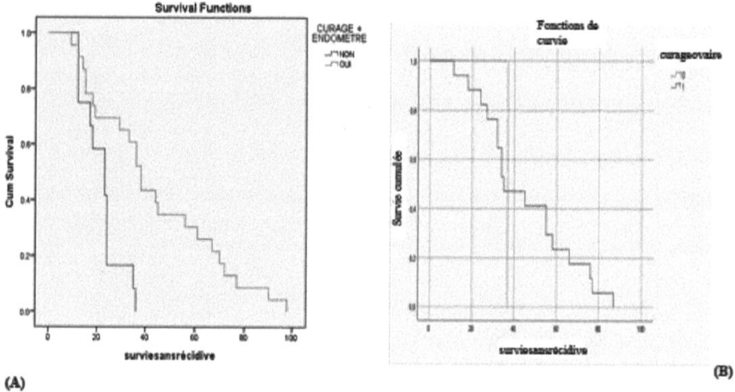

__Figure 24:__ Recurrence-free survival for endometrial cancer and ovarian cancer according to CLA stage

__Table IX:__ Comparison between CLA and no CLA group in terms of survival and recurrence by type of cancer

Type of cancer	Survival	CLA Group	Group without cleaning	Value of p
Cancer of The endometrium	Overall survival	45 months	24 months	0.38
	Survival to one year	22/23	12/12	0.46
	Survival at 2	17/23	5/12	0.06
	Survival at 3	15/23	3/12	**0.02** significant
	Relapse-free survival	38 months	23 months	**0.002** significant
	Relapse-free survival at 3 years	14/22	1/10	**0.004** significant
Cancer of ovary	Overall survival	46.65 months	37 months	0.68
	Survival at one year	15/17	1/1	0.71
	Survival at 2	13/17	1/1	0.582
	Survival at 3	11/17	1/1	0.46
	Relapse-free survival	45 months	37 months	0,72

| | Relapse-free survival at 3 years 8/14 | 1/1 | 0.6 |

CLA: lumbo-aortic curage, p: degree of significance

In terms of survival, in our series the use of CLA for endometrial cancer resulted in better 3-year survival and recurrence-free survival. However, this beneficial effect of CLA has not been demonstrated in ovarian cancer. We admit that survival in ovarian cancer could be linked to other factors that we were unable to study, in particular the absence of tumour residue during surgery.

4 DISCUSSION

1. KEY RESULTS

Our study was carried out over a period of 18 years and included 85 cases of gynaecological cancer in which lumbo-aortic curage was indicated.

For the epidemiological profile of our population, the mean age was 58.4 years [39 and 75 years]. Eleven patients (20%) had a history of gynaecological cancer. Metrorrhagia and the discovery of a pelvic mass were the most common symptoms in our series, occurring in 45.5% of cases.

The factors statistically correlated with failure to perform lumbo-aortic curage that we were able to identify were obesity, the presence of complications during pelvic curage, the type of cancer and the years of experience of the surgical team. In multivariate analysis, only the surgeon's experience and complications during pelvic resection were decisive.

We noted the presence of 30 intraoperative complications divided into grades: Grade 1 (50%), Grade 2 (26.7%), Grade 3 (20%) and Grade 4 (3.3%). There were no cases of preoperative death. It appears that CLA is associated with an increased rate of intraoperative complications, but with no significant difference for advanced grade complications.

Forty-three postoperative complications were recorded; Grade 1 (67.4%), Grade 2 (23%) and Grade 3 (9.3%). There was no difference between the curage and non-curage groups.

Recurrence was more frequent in the non-curage group. For endometrial cancer, CLA was associated with a lower rate of recurrence in the early stages. However, for endometrial cancer, the CLA procedure did not reduce the recurrence rate.

The median overall survival for our population was 38 months, i.e. 45 months in the CLA group and 36 months in the non-CLA group.

Analysis of survival by type of cancer showed that CLA significantly improved 3-year survival and recurrence-free survival in endometrial cancer.

2. STRENGTHS AND WEAKNESSES OF OUR STUDY

The key points of our study were :

■ This is a subject that has received little attention in the Tunisian literature, which makes this study all the more important, since it will enable us to study the characteristics of this pathology in our population.

■ Patients were selected over a long period spanning 18 years.

■ This is the largest series of studies carried out in Tunisia on lumbo-aortic curage.

■ We have identified several factors that limit the use of lumbo-aortic curage in pelvic gynaecological cancers.

- We analysed the descriptive results by group and also by type and stage of cancer, which enabled us to draw some conclusions.

Our study was limited by :

- Methodological limitations linked to its retrospective and monocentric nature.

- The files were sometimes missing, limiting the collection of essential data.

- Some of the patients were lost to follow-up treatment.

3. EPIDEMIOLOGICAL DATA

3.1. Patient characteristics

Eighty-five patients with gynecological cancer indicating lumbo-aortic curage were treated at Ben Arous Regional Hospital over a period of 18 years. The mean age was 58 years with extremes from 39 to 75 years. Twenty percent of the patients had a family history of gynaecological cancer and 47% and 42% respectively had a history of hypertension and diabetes.

Metrorrhagia was the most common symptom in our series (25 patients, i.e. 40%) and the average time between onset of symptoms and diagnosis of cancer was 1 month.

The epidemiological data from our study were comparable to those in the literature, in particular the study by Cartron et al in 2005 [1] and that by Imboden et al (on 279 patients) [6], whose epidemiological data are summarised in the following table in relation to our study (Table X).

Table X: Description of the population according to studies

	Our study	Cartron et al [1]	Imboden et al [6]	AbuRustum+ Dennis [7]
Number	55	915	279	100
Type of cancer	Endometrium: 33 Ovary: 20 Collar: 2	Endometrium: 178 Ovary: 98 Col : 453	Endometrium: 279 Ovary: 0 Collar: 0	Endometrium: 100 Ovary: 0 Collar: 0
Average age	58	45	62,8	58,4
BMI (kg/m)²	32,7	25,1	28,1	39,3
Nulliparitis	30,9%	-	25,7%	-
Post menopause	81,8%		87,8%	
Abdominal scar	25,5%	-	-	44,1%

BMI: body mass index

3.2. Characteristics of the procedure

3.2.1. Feasibility

The feasibility and efficacy of the CLA surgical technique in our series were comparable to those reported in the literature. The success rate was 74.5%. This rate was 79.6% for Zdenek [8] and 83% for Altgassen [9]. In Mr Cartron's study [1], carried out on a larger sample, the curage procedure failed in only 16 of the 1,102 cases, i.e. a failure rate of no more than 1.45%.

Whatever the type of gynaecological cancer treated, when lymph node dissection is indicated, it should involve the pelvic area as well as the lumbo-aortic area, given the proven risk of lumbo-aortic involvement alone in 6% of cases in the literature [3].

3.2.2. *Completion time*

3.2.2.1 Duration of the operation

The median operating time in our study was 5 hours, with extremes between 2 and 8 hours. However, the total operating time is not a reliable factor to consider, given that the nature of the surgical procedure associated with curage varies according to the type of cancer, the stage of the disease and its histological type. In the study by Deschamps [10], the mean duration of surgery was 215 minutes, with extremes between 104 and 320 minutes, whereas in the study by Mr Johnson [11], the mean duration was 310 minutes, which is in line with the results of our study.

3.2.2.2. Duration of the cleaning itself

The mean time for pelvic and lumbo-aortic curage was 119.25 minutes in the study by Altgassen et al [9], whereas the mean time was 244 minutes in the study by Imboden [6], which is in line with the results of our study with a mean of 185 minutes required for pelvic + lumbo-aortic curage by laparotomy.

In Cartron's study [1], the average duration of curage was 280 minutes for patients operated on laparoscopically.

3.2.3. *Number of lymph nodes collected*

In our study, the median number of nodes removed during curage was 28 per curage, with extremes ranging from 10 to 58 nodes, including an average of 8 lumbo-aortic nodes [2-19].

These results were much lower than in the study by Cartron [1] et al where the average number of nodes removed was 38 with 20 lumbo-aortic nodes. However, a lower rate of nodes removed on average was noted in the study by Abu Rustum [7] et al which was carried out on 114 patients over 8 years and which had an average of 10.7 nodes removed per curage including 5.7 lumbo-aortic nodes (Table XI).

For Mariani [12], a minimum of ten pelvic nodes and five lumbo-aortic nodes are sufficient, while Benedetti [13] suggests a systematic resection of at least 25 pelvic nodes and 18 lumbo-aortic nodes to consider the procedure accurate. However, these studies were based on a small number of patients and therefore do not have sufficient statistical power to suggest a number of lymph nodes that would define adequate curage.

<u>*Table XI:*</u> *Characteristics of the surgical procedure according to studies*

	Altgassen [9]	Cartron [1]	Imboden [6]	Abu Rhustum [7]	Our study
Number	59	1102	58	114	55
Feasibility	83%	97,93%	---	92%	74.5%
Duration of act op	-	-	244	250	300
Duration of cleaning	142.9	280	---	---	185
Average number of nodes removed	31	38	36	16	28
Number of positive nodes (as a percentage)	---	47%	---	21%	19%

op: operative

4. BENEFITS AND INDICATIONS OF CURAGE

4.1. The benefits of cleaning

The practice of lumbo-aortic curage in the management of gynaecological cancers is still the subject of much controversy. It is a delicate and cumbersome surgical technique requiring perfect mastery of the technique and a good knowledge of the anatomy of the pelvic-abdominal region and its variants. For pelvic cancers, LAC can be performed for the purpose of systematic staging, which targets impalpable lymph nodes, in order to determine the progression potential and extent of the disease, especially in the presence of major risk factors for lymph node involvement [14].

Dissection may also be necessary in cases of macroscopic invasion, with the aim of reducing the tumour mass [2,16,17].

The benefits of lymphadenectomy are twofold: diagnostic, because it is the most reliable technique for assessing lymph node involvement, and prognostic, because regardless of the site of the primary tumour (uterine or adnexal), the survival of patients with lymph node involvement is often poorer [2,15].

4.1.1. Ovarian cancer

The aim of lumbo-aortic and pelvic curage in ovarian cancer is twofold: accurate assessment of the stage of the disease and optimal tumour cytoreduction, which is an essential prognostic factor [2].

FIGO has been recommending surgical evaluation of pelvic and lumbo-aortic lymph node status in ovarian cancer since 1988 (Appendix 2), since lymph node involvement is frequent and poorly systematic in the early stages of the disease. It is around 14% in stage I and 28% in stage II [2, 5, 18].

A review of the literature shows that lymph node metastases are found in both the pelvic and lumbo-aortic regions without any significant correlation, and may also be contralateral to the ovarian tumour or bilateral [2]. In our series we have not noted any cases of lymph node skipping. In fact, in all cases of lumbo-aortic lymph node invasion (6 cases) there was associated pelvic lymph node invasion. The presence of lumbo-aortic lymph node metastases is of pejorative significance, since 5-year survival falls from 70% to less than 20%, independently of other prognostic factors [18-20].

Petru [22] has shown the beneficial effect of CLA on lymph node recurrence in the early stages of ovarian cancer. According to this author, failure to perform CLA increases the risk of lymph node recurrence. Better still, recurrences appear to be more likely to be peritoneal or metastatic when lumbo-aortic lymphadenectomy is performed.

In contrast, the results of the randomised trial reported by Maggioni [13] showed that 5-year recurrence-free survival and overall survival were not statistically different in the case of lymphadenectomy or selective adenectomy compared with no lymph node procedure. Furthermore, there was no difference in retro-peritoneal recurrence.

In our series, 5 patients were at an early stage. All of them had a CLA and none of them presented a recurrence.

Surgery for advanced stages is based on the importance of tumour reduction surgery [13,17-19]. In fact, in the meta-analysis by Bristow [21], each 10% reduction in the size of the tumour residue increases the median survival by 5.5%, so the current reference surgery should achieve zero tumour residue, giving a 5-year recurrence-free survival of 60%.

Several authors have noted an improvement in overall survival after CLA in advanced forms, comparing the impact of optimal or sub-optimal tumour reduction surgery, alone or combined with lymphadenectomy [13,16,18,19,21]. In a study of 13918 cases of stage III-IV ovarian cancer, Chan [22] reported a significant increase in 5-year recurrence-free survival in patients who had undergone LAC. In our study, recurrence-free survival at 3 years in advanced forms was better in the CLA group but there was no significant difference between the two groups; the tumour residue after reduction surgery could not be determined.

There are several arguments in favour of the therapeutic effect of lumbo-aortic curage. Firstly, it allows direct eradication of retro-peritoneal metastatic localisations, particularly in the early stages. Secondly, CLA allows better staging of the cancer, which in turn allows adjuvant treatment to be better adapted [16,17,21].

4.1.2. *Endometrial cancer*

In 1988, FIGO recommended surgical staging for endometrial cancer as an alternative to clinical staging, which was characterised by imprecise preoperative assessment and the absence of lymph node evaluation [3,12].

Surgical exploration remains the most accurate method for identifying lymph node metastases, enabling tumours initially classified as stage I, II, IIIa and IIIb to be reclassified as stage IIIc. In a study of 1109 patients with clinical stage I and II tumours, Benedetti showed that lymph node metastases were present in 11% of cases [23]. Creasman studied the risk of lymph node metastases in 621 women with clinical stage I and II. He found that the risk was 11%: 9% pelvic and 6% lumbo-aortic [24]. In our series, the rate of lymph node metastases for all stages combined was 26%, and in a third of cases the cancer was at an early stage.

Attitudes are highly controversial on both sides of the Atlantic. The American recommendations advocate broad indications for LAM, whereas the European school recommends LAM only in the presence of risk factors for lymph node metastases. Surgical lymph node staging should currently be performed in patients with high-risk or intermediate-high-risk disease [3].

Sentinel lymph node biopsy is an acceptable alternative to systematic lymphadenectomy for lymph node staging in stages I/II [3, 8,14]. Indeed, to compensate for total lymphadenectomy, which remains a major surgical procedure, the learned societies currently recommend the use of this sentinel lymph node technique [3,6,12].

Although CLA seems necessary for staging, its impact on survival, which is a decisive factor in definitively validating its indication, remains to be demonstrated [22].

In the early stages, its contribution to overall survival and recurrence-free survival has been shown in several studies to be of no benefit. According to Kadar, 108 CLAs are required to save one life [25]. Trimble, in a study of 9185 stage I patients, reported a relative improvement in survival for high-grade tumours [26].

In a large retrospective study of 12333 patients, Chan [22] found no significant benefit for low-risk tumours. On the other hand, he observed an increase in 5-year survival in high-risk patients who had undergone LAC, from 76.3 to 81.7% for grade 3 stage Ic and from 82.2 to 90.4% for stage II.

In contrast, several studies such as those by Togami [15] and Eltabbakh [27] showed better survival in patients who had undergone lymphadenectomy. Similarly, in our study, better overall and recurrence-free survival was observed in the CLA group in the early stages of the disease.

Havrilesky studied the impact of CLA in advanced stages (IIIC) of endometrial cancer. According to this author, leaving macroscopically involved lymph nodes reduces survival. Indeed, the 5-year survival in patients with microscopic involvement and those with macroscopic involvement treated by complete lymphadenectomy was 63 and 50% respectively, whereas it was 43% if residual macroscopic involvement remained [28].

Fujimoto, in a population of 63 stage IIIc patients, found a recurrence-free survival of 53.9% compared with 69.1% in the case of complete lomboaortic lymphadenectomy combined with pelvic lymphadenectomy [29].

Mariani [12] and Chan [22] found a benefit to lymphadenectomy on 5-year survival for stage III or IV patients which was significantly related to the number of lymph nodes removed.

4.1.3. *Cervical cancer*

Node involvement is a major prognostic factor in cervical cancer. The survival rate in stage I is between 80% and 98%, falling to less than 50% in the presence of lymph node metastases [30-32].

Lumbo-aortic lymph nodes are not considered regional lymph nodes. Invasion of these lymph nodes results in the disease being classified as metastatic stage IVB. The relative risk of death in cases of lumbo-aortic involvement is estimated at between 4.66 and 6 [30-32].

Lumbo-aortic dissection is thought to have a therapeutic effect by allowing adjuvant or neoadjuvant treatment to be adapted according to its results. Extending the field of irradiation (combined with chemotherapy) improves survival in cases of lumbo-aortic metastases [33,34].

Surgical sampling is the gold standard for the detection of lymph node involvement in the early stages. Indeed, pelvic lymphadenectomy is part of the surgical procedure for the management of early-stage cervical cancer [31,33,35]. However, its therapeutic value is not well understood, although radiotherapy alone, even if it provides the same results in terms of survival, would be more morbid than LAC [31,33,36].

The standard treatment for locally advanced cervical cancer (stages Ib2, IIA >4 cm, IIb, III and IVA and/or in the presence of lymph node metastases) is currently based on concomitant neoadjuvant chemo-radiotherapy with or without brachytherapy [30,31,36]. This approach has now been validated, confirming the benefit of chemotherapy including cisplatin [32,37].

Removal of metastatic lumbo-aortic nodes appears to have an impact on patient survival [35,39]. Marnitz [34] reported that removal of more than 5 metastatic lombo-aortic lymph nodes was associated with an increase in the recurrence-free survival rate. He also noted that after CLA the survival rate was similar in patients with lymph node invasion and those without lymph node invasion.

Holcomb, in a retrospective study of 274 patients with stages IIB to IVA, found a significant improvement in survival [38].

At present, given the morbidity associated with adjuvant radiotherapy and the difficulty of performing surgery on the CLA after the initial radio-chemotherapy, several authors are proposing laparoscopic pre-therapy staging [35,39, 40]. In 2013, Gouy highlighted the prospect of minimally invasive surgery using an extra-peritoneal approach in locally advanced cervical cancer, demonstrating its feasibility and the gain in terms of survival in the PET-CT era when integrated with radio-chemotherapy with extension of the radiation fields in the case of metastatic lumbo-aortic adenopathy [39].

4.2. Indications for CLA in pelvic gynecological cancers

✓ In ovarian cancer, CLA is essential during the initial surgery with a view to complete resection (zero residue). If this objective cannot be achieved during the initial surgery, additional lymph node re-staging may be considered as an option during interval surgery after neoadjuvant chemotherapy [3,16].

✓ In endometrial cancer, surgical lymph node staging should be performed in patients with high-risk or intermediate high-risk disease and in type 2 endometrial cancers. Conversely, systematic lymphadenectomy is not recommended in the low and intermediate risk group. Sentinel lymph node biopsy may be considered for staging in patients in this group. It is not recommended for patients without myometrial invasion in this group [3].

When a systematic lymphadenectomy is carried out, pelvic and para-aortic infra-renal lymph node dissection is suggested. Lymph node dissection is a staging procedure that allows adjuvant treatment to be adapted [3,40].

✓ In cervical cancer, there is no consensus regarding lumbo-aortic curage [30,31].

For stages less than Ib2, pelvic curage is of prime importance in guiding adjuvant treatment. Lumbo-aortic curage is performed if pelvic curage is positive [30].

For stages Ib2, Iia, IIb, III and IVa, the reference treatment is concomitant radio-chemotherapy. Lumbo-aortic dissection is indicated as an option, best performed with PET scans and minimally invasive surgery [31,41].

5. LIMITS TO CLEANING LUMBO-AORTIC

5.1. Age and co-morbidities

At present, there is no solid evidence to suggest that age is a limiting factor in lumbo-aortic curage. In fact, age and comorbidities have been little studied in the literature, and only a few studies have addressed these two parameters. Mariani [12] and Benedetti [42] suspected the presence of age-related comorbidities as a factor that could either derail the curage procedure because of an intraoperative complication or encourage laparoscopic conversion when curage was started laparoscopically.

In the recent study by Asa Akesson, age and the presence of comorbidities did not significantly increase the rate of complications during pelvic and lumbo-aortic curage [43].

For our study, there was no significant difference in age between the two CLEs and without CLA, and this factor was not retained as a determining factor limiting the use of CLAs.

5.2. Body mass index

In 2001, Scribner [44] presented the largest series of "obese" patients treated by laparoscopy. He reported that obesity appeared to be the only factor limiting lumbo-aortic curage, particularly that performed laparoscopically. Cartron's study also confirmed that obesity is the main factor in the failure of lumbo-aortic curage procedures [1]. In the Ucella study [45], the success rate fell from 82.1% for a BMI of less than 35 to 44.4% for a BMI of more than 35.

The recent study by Asa Akesson [43] showed that a BMI value greater than 30 was significantly associated with an increased rate of intraoperative complications during pelvic and lumbo-aortic curage.

In our study we found no significant difference in BMI between the two groups (p=0.02) with an area under the curve equal to 0.77 and a threshold value of 34. Furthermore, we found that above a BMI value of 34, the risk of failure of lumbo-aortic curage was greater, with a significant difference (p=0.03).

5.3. Presence of fixed lymph nodes

In the studies by Dargent [46], Chapron [47] and Cartron [1], the presence of fixed lymph nodes during lumbo-aortic curage was one of the main factors in procedure failure or laparoconversion when curage was planned by crelioscopy, but the rate was only 1 to 2% in the different series. However, this remains an old notion that is tending to disappear in the new series due to the training of surgical teams and the progress made in radiology, which allows macroscopically suspicious lymph nodes to be identified on CT or MRI and biopsied for histological proof [28]. In our series, this detail was not mentioned in the operative reports, particularly in the case of failed CLA.

5.4. Adherences

In Abu Rustum's study of 204 patients, only 8% required laparoscopic curage to be stopped due to the presence of solid adhesions, out of a total failure rate of 43.6% for lumbo-aortic curage procedures [9].

In our study, the failure rate due to the presence of solid adhesions was 5.45%. The difference between the two groups was not significant (p=0.465) and we did not consider this factor to be a limiting factor for performing CLA, at least by laparotomy.

5.5. Complications during pelvic curage

Several studies have shown that pelvic curage alone, particularly when performed by laparotomy, increases the risk of per-operative complications. In the multicentre study by Palomba et al [48] on 1174 patients with operable endometrial cancer, it was shown that the occurrence of complications during pelvic curage was responsible for 8 cases of failure of the curage procedure, although this was not statistically significant. Similarly, in the studies by Dargent [46] and Asa Akesson [43], complications of pelvic curage did not significantly increase the failure rate of lumbo-aortic curage. Conversely, in our series, the occurrence of these complications was related to the risk of failure of lumbo-aortic curage. After multi-variate analysis, we retained this factor as a determinant of the success or failure of CLA.

5.6. Operator experience

Seventy-five per cent of the intraoperative vascular complications leading to failure of the CLA procedure occurred in the first half of the series of pelvic and lumbo-aortic lymphadenectomies in Cartron's study [1]. Chapron studied the role of the surgeon's experience in the success of CLA in three studies. This author insists that the experience acquired by the surgeon significantly reduces the number of per-operative complications during curage. This number fell from 4.86/1000 to 2.36/1000. With years of surgical experience, technical progress has been made, particularly in adhesiolysis techniques, thus reducing the number of digestive lesions [49-51].

Our study also showed that the experience of the surgical team played a major role, not only in achieving a complete and exhaustive lumbo-aortic curage, but also in terms of the number of complications preventing this curage from being carried out. The median years of experience was 14 years for the CLA group compared with 7 years for the group without curage, with a significant difference between the two groups (p = 0.04).

5.7. Type of cancer

In the literature, the type of cancer treated was not a factor influencing lumbo-aortic curage, whatever the surgical technique [1,6,48]. In our study, although we found a significant difference between endometrial cancer and ovarian cancer in the univariate study, this factor was not retained in the multivariate study (Table XII).

Table XII: Factors limiting the success of CLA

Author	Year	Number of cases	Age/ morbidity	Obesite	Adherence fixes	Gg	Complications during pelvic curage	Experience of the operator	Type of cancer
Dargent [46]	2000	40						+	
Kohler [52]	2004	606		+					

Cartron [1]	2005	915		-		-		
Ee [53]	2018	100	-		-			
Akesson [43]	2021	556	-	+		+	-	
Ourstudy	2022	55	-	+	--	+	+	+

gg: ganglion

6. COMPLICATIONS OF LUMBO-AORTIC CURAGE

6.1. Morbidity (Table XIII)

6.1.1. Length of stay

The results of our study concerning the length of hospitalisation were not consistent with the literature, with an average of 25 days, whereas the average number of days of hospitalisation was between 2 and 5 days [1,9,44,48].

6.1.2. Duration of the act

The curage is associated with an extension of the operating time of between one and three hours, with an average extension of 1h,10 min in our series. The same applies to all the series in the literature, with an average of between 250-300 minutes for the surgical procedure as a whole, the operating time specific to the curage itself being between 130 and 180 min [1,5,49-51].

6.1.3. Stay in intensive care

In our series, only one patient was transferred to intensive care. This concept remains unclear in the literature, since all the studies were carried out in hospitals run by a trained resuscitation team.

Table XIII: Morbidity according to studies

Morbidity	Asa Akesson [43]	Imboden [6]	Our study
Number of patients	549	279	55
Length of hospital stay (average)	2-3	4	28
Stay in intensive care	-	-	1.8%
Duration of operation (in hours)	250-300 min	244 min	280 min
Duration of cleaning (average)	134 min	121 min	185 min
Transfusion	35	---	6
Blood loss	-	240 ml	----

avg: average, min: minute, ml: millilitres.

6.2. Complications of curage

6.2.1. Intraoperative complications

6.2.1.1. Number of complications

The use of the new classification published in the British Medical Journal in 2020 has changed the perspective for estimating the number of complications and their grades, particularly in major surgery such as that for pelvic gynaecological cancers [4]. As a result, there is a wide discrepancy between the results found in the largest series of lumbo-aortic curage in the literature.

A low rate of intraoperative complications in CLA has been reported in studies by Cartron and Imboden, with rates of 1.96% and 2.5% respectively [1,55].

Conversely, high rates of up to 31% have been found in the literature [2,46,48,53-61].

In our study, the rate of intraoperative complications was 26.8%. This rate was equal to that reported by d'Akesson in 2021 [43]. The results of our study concur with those of this author on the fact that CLA significantly increases the rate of intraoperative complications.

6.2.1.2. Grade of intraoperative complications

For grade 1 complications, our results are in line with the literature, and it appears that CLA does not increase this type of complication.

For the other grades, the literature is divided. Our results concur with those reported by Imboden [6] and Abu Rostum [7] that CLA does not increase complications of grade 2 and above. Conversely, Akesson showed in his study that these types of complications were correlated with CLA [43] (Table XIV).

Table XIV: Number and grade of intraoperative complications according to studies

	Abu Rustum [7]	Akesson [43]	Imboden [6]	Our study
Number of patients	114	549	279	55
Number of complications	8	143	7	30
Complications in the CLA group	8	103	58	18
Complications in the Failure group	0	446	103	12
Complication Grade 1	7	35	4	15
Value of p	NS	NS	NS	0.74
Complication Grade 2, 3, 4	1	108	3	15
Value of p	NS	< 0,001	NS	NS

CLA: lumbo-aortic curage, NS: not significant, p: degree of significance

6.2.2. Post-operative complications

6.2.2.1. Grade 1 complications

■ Wall abscess was present in 7 cases in our study, with no difference between the two groups. These results were similar to those found in the literature [9,43,62-64].

■ Prolonged ileus was noted in 8 cases, only one of which was related to a radiologically confirmed intestinal obstruction managed by conservative treatment. This rate was similar to that found in the various series, varying between 0 and 3 cases [1,43,57,59,60]. The difference between the CLA group and the group without curage was not significant, as were the data in the literature.

6.2.2.2. Grade 2 complications

■ Thromboembolic complications occurred in 4 cases, all in the CLA group. This number varied according to the different series, ranging from 1 to 3 [9,43,58]. We found no significant difference between the two groups. Conversely, Akesson showed that this type of complication was correlated with CLA [43].

■ In Cartron's study [1] of 915 patients, five required a blood transfusion, all of whom were CLA. In our series, blood transfusion was required for 6 patients, five of whom were CLA, so curage significantly increased the risk of blood transfusion. These results are in line with those of Akesson [43] and Imboden [62].

6.2.2.3. Lymphocele

Lymphoceles are the most frequent postoperative complication of pelvic and lumbo-aortic lymphadenectomy, varying from 0.5 to 58% depending on the series, but rarely complicated [1,59,65-68]. The exact rate of lymphoceles remains difficult to assess in our series because there was no systematic radiological screening. Only symptomatic lymphoceles were reported and treated.

Symptomatic lymphocele was found in 11 cases in our series: 10 in the CLA group and 1 in the group without curage, with no significant difference between the two groups. Lumbo-aortic curage appears to be associated with a higher rate of symptomatic lymphocele, but not to a statistically significant extent, which is in line with the results found in the literature [1,59,65-68] (Table XV).

Table XV: Number of postoperative complications "CLA" VS "without CLA".

	Abces of the wall	Ileus	Thromboembolic complications	Transfusion	Lymphocele
Akesson [43]	NS	-	P<0,002	P<0,002	-
Cartron [1]	NS	---	NS	---	NS
Panici [42]	-	NS	-	P=0,006	-
Rahm [65]	P=0,01	---	---	---	NS
Our series	4/3 (NS)	7/1(NS)	4/0(NS)	5/1 NS	10/1 NS

NS: not significant, p: significance level

7. PROGNOSIS OF PATIENTS TREATED WITH LUMBO-AORTIC CURAGE

7.1. Ovarian cancer

The trial by Magionni et al [13] compared a group with lymphadenectomy and another without lymphadenectomy in early stage ovarian cancer (stages I-II). Lymph node surgery did not appear to have a statistically significant impact on the overall survival of patients in this trial, although there was a trend towards improved survival in those who underwent complete lymph node surgery. One of the explanations given in the study's conclusion is the lack of power, due to the probably insufficient numbers to show a significant difference.

In our series, we had 18 cases of ovarian cancer, 73% of which were at an advanced stage. The cases treated at a limited pelvic stage (I-II) all belonged to the CLA group and had an overall survival rate of 47.4 months. There was only one case of recurrence (1/3) at this stage.

These results were in line with those found in the literature and could be explained by complete lymph node surgery increasing the overall survival rate and reducing the risk of local recurrence [18,19,42]. Chambers conducted the first randomised trial of the therapeutic impact of lumbo-aortic curage in advanced ovarian cancer, demonstrating that there was a benefit to complete lymph node surgery in terms of recurrence-free survival.

However, the lack of impact of this systematic surgery on overall patient survival has led to the conclusion that complete lymphadenectomy in advanced stage ovarian cancer should be abandoned [21,34,42]. In recent studies, in particular the study by Gouy [2], the gain in survival between patients with a millimetre-sized remnant (less than 5 mm) at the end of of surgery and those who had macroscopically complete surgery (no visible remnant) is sufficiently evocative to define the latter surgery as a standard, involving both intra- and retro-peritoneal lymphadenectomy. The impact of CLA on the patients in our series was marked by a considerable improvement in terms of overall survival (46.6 months vs 37) and recurrence-free survival (45 months vs 37), but this difference was not statistically significant.

7.2. Endometrial cancer

The therapeutic value of a complete, bilateral pelvic lymphadenectomy extending to the lomboaortic region has been suggested in N+ patients in terms of overall survival and recurrence-free survival. Large studies conclude that there is a positive correlation between the number of lymph nodes removed and overall survival [1,23,28,29,39].

The therapeutic value of CLA was also studied by Fujimoto et al [29] in their series of 63 patients (stage IIIC) divided into two groups according to whether or not CLA was performed. No significant difference in survival was found between the two groups. On the other hand, there was a survival benefit in patients receiving a PTA if the number of invaded pelvic lymph nodes was greater than or equal to 2. The series by Mariani et al [12], involving 51 stage IIIC patients following the same schema, found a benefit in favour of the CLA group. The authors noted the absence of recurrence in 85% of patients treated with pelvic and lumbo-aortic lymphadenectomy followed by adjuvant radiotherapy.

In our study, lumbo-aortic curage showed a statistically significant gain in terms of overall survival and recurrence-free survival. Similarly, the recurrence rate was much better for the CLA group (4.3% vs 16.6%) in localised cancers. Our results are in line with those of Mariani.

7.3. Cervical cancer

In the case of lumbo-aortic metastases of cervical cancer, the prognosis is very favourable. Overall survival is 28% at 3 years, and recurrence-free survival is 15% in stages IB2-II. For the same stages without lumbo-aortic involvement, these survival rates are 88% and 74% respectively [11,21,34,39]. In view of the very poor survival results in cases of lumbo-aortic involvement detected at "closure", lymphadenectomy does not appear to be justified at the end of treatment after radio-chemotherapy [11,38,41].

Our series included two patients aged 55 and 45 with stage IB1 cervical cancer, one of whom had undergone lumbo-aortic curage and had better overall and recurrence-free survival than the group without CLA. Recurrence was noted at 17 months for the patient in the non-CLA group despite a good initial response to concomitant radio-chemotherapy (Figure 25).

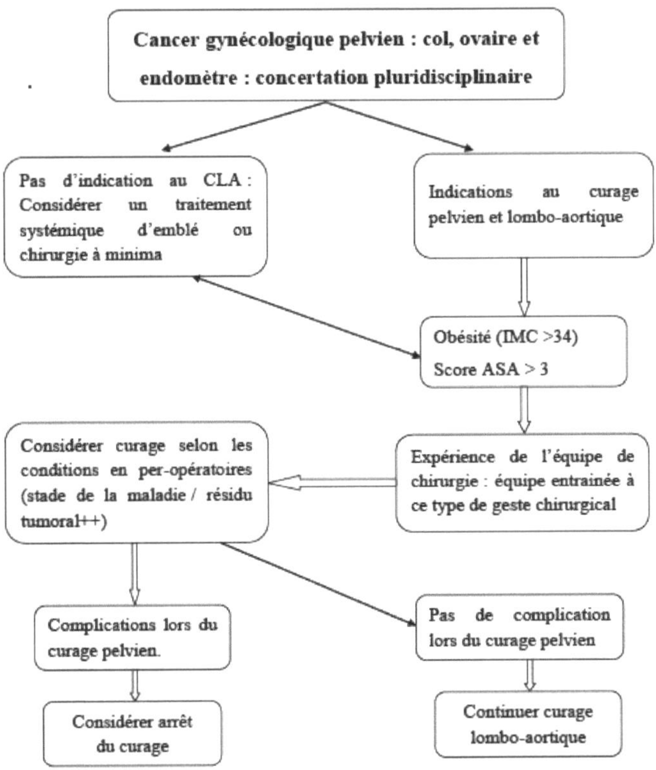

Pelvic gynaecological cancer: cervix, ovary and endometrium:

multidisciplinary consultation

No indication for CLA: consider immediate systemic treatment or minimally invasive surgery

Indications for pelvic and lumbo-aortic curage

Obesity (BMI >34) ASA score > 3

Experience of the surgical team: team trained in this type of surgical procedure

Consider curage depending on intra-operative conditions (stage of disease / tumour residue++)

Complications during pelvic curage.

No complications during pelvic curage

Consider stopping cleaning

Continue lumbo-aortic curage

***Figure 25:** Flow chart for the management of patients with gynecologicalpelvic cancer with or without indication for lumbo-aortic curage cancer with or without indication for lumbo-aortic curage*

5 CONCLUSION

Lumbo-aortic curage (LAC) is not a trivial procedure, and the question of its prognostic and therapeutic value needs to be addressed. Its indication should be systematically discussed at a multi-disciplinary consultation meeting. The operating technique is now perfectly codified, but this procedure is associated with specific morbidity and an increased rate of intra- and post-operative complications.

In order to determine the benefits, limitations and possible complications of this surgical technique, we conducted a retrospective study including 85 patients operated on for pelvic gynecological cancer with curative intent, over a 19-year period from January 2003 to December 2021, in the obstetric gynecology department of the Ben Arous regional hospital.

The aim of our work was to study the epidemiological and clinical profile of patients, to clarify the indications and limitations of lumbo-aortic curage, and to describe the intra- and post-operative complications in order to determine the current place of this technique in the treatment of gynaecological cancers.

In our series, the factors associated with the failure to perform lumbo-aortic curage in the univariate study were the type of cancer, obesity, the occurrence of complications during pelvic curage and the experience of the surgeon. In the multivariate study, only the experience of the surgical team and the presence of complications during pelvic curage were independent factors in the failure to perform lumbo-aortic curage.

Our comparative study also showed that lumbo-aortic curage was responsible for a significant increase in operating time and in the number of intraoperative complications, without having any impact on the severity of these complications. Better still, no significant increase in the number or grade of complications was reported postoperatively.

In terms of survival, CLA for endometrial cancer resulted in improved 3-year survival and recurrence-free survival for patients. However, this beneficial effect of CLA has not been demonstrated in ovarian cancer.

Concerning the study of recurrence, CLA was associated with a lower rate of recurrence in the early stages of endometrial cancer. However, the occurrence of recurrence of ovarian cancer was not related to whether or not CLA was performed. Recurrence was more frequent in advanced forms.

Lumbo-aortic curettage therefore takes on its full diagnostic, therapeutic and prognostic importance for endometrial cancers when it is indicated. For ovarian cancer, which is often diagnosed at an advanced stage of the disease, LAC must be performed on a case-by-case basis depending on the stage and type of cancer, the surgeon's experience and the estimated tumour residue at the end of surgery.

Finally, we would like to emphasise the value of multidisciplinary consultation in the case of pelvic gynaecological cancer, in order to determine the correct indication for lumbo-aortic curage, taking into account the balance between the therapeutic benefit of carcinology and the risk of peri-operative morbidity and mortality.

6 REFERENCES

[1] Cartron G, Leblanc E, Ferron G, Martel P, Narducci F, Querleu D. [Complications of laparoscopic lymphadenectomy in gynaecologic oncology. A series of 1102 procedures in 915 patients]. Gynecol Obstet Fertil 2005;33:304-14.

[2] Gouy S. Are there still indications for lumboaortic curage in gynaecological cancers in 2008? Yes, and more than ever... - Place of para-aortic lymphadenectomy in gynecological cancers in 2008. 2008:4.

[3] Concin N, Matias-Guiu X, Vergote I, Cibula D, Mirza MR, Marnitz S, et al. ESGO/ESTRO/ESP guidelines for the management of patients with endometrial carcinoma. Int J Gynecol Cancer Off J Int Gynecol Cancer Soc 2021;31:12-39.

[4] Dell-Kuster S, Gomes NV, Gawria L, Aghlmandi S, Aduse-Poku M, Bissett I, et al. Prospective validation of classification of intraoperative adverse events (ClassIntra): international, multicentre cohort study. BMJ 2020;370:m2917.

[5] Querleu D, Lanvin D, Elhage A, Henry-Buisson B, Leblanc E. An objective experimental assessment of the learning curve for laparoscopic surgery: the example of pelvic and para-aortic lymph node dissection. Eur J Obstet Gynecol Reprod Biol 1998;81:55-8.

[6] Imboden S, Mereu L, Siegenthaler F, Pellegrini A, Papadia A, Tateo S, et al. Oncological safety and perioperative morbidity in low-risk endometrial cancer with sentinel lymph-node dissection. Eur J Surg Oncol 2019;45:1638-43.

[7] Abu-Rustum NR, Chi DS, Sonoda Y, DiClemente MJ, Bekker G, Gemignani M, et al. Transperitoneal laparoscopic pelvic and para-aortic lymph node dissection using the argon-beam coagulator and monopolar instruments: an 8-year study and description of technique. Gynecol Oncol 2003;89:504-13.

[8] Holub Z, Jabor A, Bartos P, Hendl J, Urbanek S. Laparoscopic surgery in women with endometrial cancer: the learning curve. Eur J Obstet Gynecol Reprod Biol 2003;107:195-200.

[9] Altgassen C. Establishing a new technique of laparoscopic pelvic and para-aortic lymphadenectomy. Obstet Gynecol 2000;95:348-52.

[10] Deschamps C, Allen MS, Trastek VF, Johnson JO, Pairolero PC. Early experience and learning curve associated with laparoscopic Nissen fundoplication. J Thorac Cardiovasc Surg 1998;115:281-5.

[11] Johnson N. Laparoscopic versus conventional pelvic lymphadenectomy for gynaecological malignancy in humans. Br J Obstet Gynaecol 1994;101:902-4.

[12] Mariani A, El-Nashar SA, Dowdy SC. Lymphadenectomy in Endometrial Cancer: Which Is the Right Question? Int J Gynecol Cancer 2010;20:S52-4.

[13] Maggioni A, Benedetti Panici P, Dell'Anna T, Landoni F, Lissoni A, Pellegrino A, et al. Randomised study of systematic lymphadenectomy in patients with epithelial ovarian cancer macroscopically confined to the pelvis. Br J Cancer 2006;95:699-704.

[14] Salhi Y, Gaillard T, Huchon C, Mezzadri M, Marchand E, Cornelis F, et al. Lumbo-aortic curage and pelvic gynecological cancers: retroperitoneal or transperitoneal crelioscopy? Gynecologic' Obstétrique Fertil Sénologie 2021;49:838-43.

[15] Togami S, Kawamura T, Fukuda M, Yanazume S, Kamio M, Kobayashi H. Learning curve and surgical outcomes for laparoscopic surgery, including pelvic lymphadenectomy, for early stage endometrial cancer. Jpn J Clin Oncol 2019;49:521-4.

[16] Lavoue V, Huchon C, Akladios C, Alfonsi P, Bakrin N, Ballester M, et al. Management of epithelial ovarian cancer. Short text drafted from the French joint recommendations of FRANCOGYN, CNGOF, SFOG, GINECO-ARCAGY and endorsed by INCa. Bull Cancer (Paris) 2019;106:354-70.

[17]Gao J, Yang X, Zhang Y. Systematic lymphadenectomy in the treatment of epithelial ovarian cancer: a meta-analysis of multiple epidemiology studies. Jpn J Clin Oncol 2015;45:49-60.

[18]Onda T, Yoshikawa H, Yasugi T, Mishima M, Nakagawa S, Yamada M, et al. Patients with ovarian carcinoma upstaged to Stage III after systematic lymphadenectomy have similar survival to Stage I/II patients and superior survival to other Stage III patients. Cancer 1998;83:1555-60.

[19]Zhou J, Shan G, Chen Y. The effect of lymphadenectomy on survival and recurrence in patients with ovarian cancer: a systematic review and meta-analysis. Jpn J Clin Oncol 2016;46:718-26.

[20]Petru E, Lahousen M, Tamussino K, Pickel H, Stranzl H, Stettner H, et al. Lymphadenectomy in stage I ovarian cancer. Am J Obstet Gynecol 1994;170:656-62.

[21]Bristow RE, Tomacruz RS, Armstrong DK, Trimble EL, Montz FJ. Survival effect of maximal cytoreductive surgery for advanced ovarian carcinoma during the platinum era: a meta-analysis. J Clin Oncol Off J Am Soc Clin Oncol 2002;20:1248-59.

[22]Chan JK, Cheung MK, Huh WK, Osann K, Husain A, Teng NN, et al. Therapeutic role of lymph node resection in endometrioid corpus cancer: a study of 12,333 patients. Cancer 2006;107:1823-30.

[23]Benedetti-Panici P, Maneschi F, Cutillo G, D'Andrea G, Manci N, Rabitti C et al. Anatomical and pathological study of retroperitoneal nodes in endometrial cancer. Int J Gynecol Cancer, 1998;8:322-327.

[24]Creasman WT, Morrow CP, Bundy BN, Homesley HD, Graham JE, Heller PB. Surgical pathologic spread patterns of endometrial cancer. A Gynecologic Oncology Group Study. Cancer 1987;60:2035-41.

[25]Kadar N. Laparoscopic pelvic and aortic lymphadenectomy. Baillieres Clin Obstet Gynaecol 1995;9:651-73.

[26]Trimble EL, Kosary C, Park RC. Lymph node sampling and survival in endometrial cancer. Gynecol Oncol 1998;71:340-3.

[27]Eltabbakh GH. Analysis of survival after laparoscopy in women with endometrial carcinoma. Cancer 2002;95:1894-901.

[28]Havrilesky LJ, Kulasingam SL, Matchar DB, Myers ER. FDG-PET for management of cervical and ovarian cancer. Gynecol Oncol 2005;97:183-91.

[29]Fujimoto T, Nanjyo H, Nakamura A, Yokoyama Y, Takano T, Shoji T, et al. Paraaortic lymphadenectomy may improve disease-related survival in patients with multipositive pelvic lymph node stage IIIc endometrial cancer. Gynecol Oncol 2007;107:253-9.

[30]Olawaiye AB, Baker TP, Washington MK, Mutch DG. The new (Version 9) American Joint Committee on Cancer tumor, node, metastasis staging for cervical cancer. CA Cancer J Clin 2021;71:287-98.

[31]Hill EK. Updates in Cervical Cancer Treatment. Clin Obstet Gynecol 2020;63:3-11.

[32]Delpech Y, Meder C, Rey A, Zafrani Y, Uzan C, Gouy S, et al. Para-Aortic Involvement and Interest of Para-Aortic Lymphadenectomy after Chemoradiation Therapy in Patients with Stage IB2 and II Cervical Carcinoma Radiologically Confined to the Pelvic Cavity. Ann Surg Oncol, 2007;14(11):3223-31.

[33]D^az-Feijo6 B, Acosta U, Toтё A, Gil-Ibanez B, Hernandez A, Domingo S, et al. Surgical Outcomes of Laparoscopic Pelvic Lymph Node Debulking during Staging Aortic Lymphadenectomy in Locally Advanced Cervical Cancer: A Multicenter Study. Cancers

2022;14.

[34] Marnitz S, Kohler C, Roth C, Fuller J, Hinkelbein W, Schneider A. Is there a benefit of pretreatment laparoscopic transperitoneal surgical staging in patients with advanced cervical cancer? Gynecol Oncol 2005;99:536-44.

[35] Mergui J-L, Polena V, David-Montefiore E, Uzan S. [Guidelines for the follow-up of women treated for high-grade cervical neoplasia]. J Gynecol Obstet Biol Reprod (Paris) 2008;37 Suppl 1:S121-130.

[36] Bhatla N, Aoki D, Sharma DN, Sankaranarayanan R. Cancer of the cervix uteri: 2021 update. Int J Gynaecol Obstet Off Organ Int Fed Gynaecol Obstet 2021;155 Suppl 1:28-44.

[37] Peters WA, Liu PY, Barret RJ, Stock RJ, Monk BJ, Berek JS et al. Concurrent Chemotherapy and Pelvic Radiation Therapy Compared with pelvic radiation therapy alone as adjuvant therapy after radical surgery in high-risk early-stage cancer of the cervix. J. Clin Oncol. 2000;18(8):1606-13.

[38] Holcomb K, Abulafia O, Matthews RP, Gabbur N, Lee YC, Buhl A. The impact of pretreatment staging laparotomy on survival in locally advanced cervical carcinoma. Eur J Gynaecol Oncol 1999;20:90-3.

[39] Sëbastien Gouy. Extraperitoneal and single-port lumbo-aortic lymphadënectomy.
in locally advanced cervical cancer: feasibility, reproducibility, ergonomic aspects and survival benefit a Гère of positron emission tomography (PET) coupled with computed tomography (CT). Medecine humaine et pathologie. Universite de Lorraine, 2013;2013LORR0095.

[40] Querleu D, Planchamp F, Chiva L, Fotopoulou C, Barton D, Cibula D, et al. European Society of Gynaecological Oncology (ESGO) Guidelines for Ovarian Cancer Surgery. Int J Gynecol Cancer Off J Int Gynecol Cancer Soc 2017;27:1534-42.

[41] Morice P, Narducci F, Mathevet P, Marret H, Darai E, Querleu D, et al. French recommendations on the management of invasive cervical cancer during pregnancy. Int J Gynecol Cancer Off J Int Gynecol Cancer Soc 2009;19:1638-41.

[42] Panici PB, Maggioni A, Hacker N, Landoni F, Ackermann S, Campagnutta E, et al. Systematic aortic and pelvic lymphadenectomy versus resection of bulky nodes only in optimally debulked advanced ovarian cancer: a randomized clinical trial. J Natl Cancer Inst 2005;97:560-6.

[43] Akesson A, Wolmesjo N, Adok C, Milsom I, Dahm-Kahler P. Lymphadenectomy, obesity and open surgery are associated with surgical complications in endometrial cancer. Eur J Surg Oncol J Eur Soc Surg Oncol Br Assoc Surg Oncol 2021;47:2907-14.

[44] Scribner DR, Walker JL, Johnson GA, McMeekin SD, Gold MA, Mannel RS. Laparoscopic pelvic and paraaortic lymph node dissection: analysis of the first 100 cases. Gynecol Oncol 2001;82:498-503.

[45] Uccella S, Bonzini M, Palomba S, Fanfani F, Ceccaroni M, Seracchioli R, et al. Impact of Obesity on Surgical Treatment for Endometrial Cancer: A Multicenter Study Comparing Laparoscopy vs Open Surgery, with Propensity-Matched Analysis. J Minim Invasive Gynecol 2016;23:53-61.

[46] Dargent D, Ansquer Y, Mathevet P. Technical development and results of left extraperitoneal laparoscopic paraaortic lymphadenectomy for cervical cancer. Gynecol Oncol 2000;77:87-92.

[47] Chapron C, Pierre F, Querleu D, Dubuisson JB. Major vascular complications of gynaecological laparoscopy. Gynecol Obstet Fertil 2000;28:880-7.

[48] Palomba S, Ghezzi F, Falbo A, Mandato VD, Annunziata G, Lucia E, et al. Conversion in endometrial cancer patients scheduled for laparoscopic staging: a large multicenter analysis: conversions and endometrial cancer. Surg Endosc 2014;28:3200-9.

[49] Chapron CM, Pierre F, Lacroix S, Querleu D, Lansac J, Dubuisson JB. Major vascular injuries during gynecologic laparoscopy. J Am Coll Surg 1997;185:461-5.

[50] Chapron C, Querleu D, Bruhat MA, Madelenat P, Fernandez H, Pierre F, et al. Surgical complications of diagnostic and operative gynaecological laparoscopy: a series of 29,966 cases. Hum Reprod Oxf Engl 1998;13:867-72.

[51] Chapron C, Pierre F, Harchaoui Y, Lacroix S, Beguin S, Querleu D, et al. Gastrointestinal injuries during gynaecological laparoscopy. Hum Reprod Oxf Engl 1999;14:333-7.

[52] Kohler C, Klemm P, Schau A, Possover M, Krause N, Tozzi R, et al. Introduction of transperitoneal lymphadenectomy in a gynecologic oncology center: analysis of 650 laparoscopic pelvic and/or paraaortic transperitoneal lymphadenectomies. Gynecol Oncol 2004;95:52-61.

[53] Ee WW, Nellore V, McMullen W, Ragupathy K. Laparoscopic hysterectomy for endometrial cancer: impact of age on clinical outcomes. J Obstet Gynaecol J Inst Obstet Gynaecol 2018;38:734.

[54] Casarin J, Multinu F, Ubl DS, Dowdy SC, Cliby WA, Glaser GE, et al. Adoption of Minimally Invasive Surgery and Decrease in Surgical Morbidity for Endometrial Cancer Treatment in the United States. Obstet Gynecol 2018;131:304-11.

[55] Spirtos NM, Eisenkop SM, Schlaerth JB, Ballon SC. Laparoscopic radical hysterectomy (type III) with aortic and pelvic lymphadenectomy in patients with stage I cervical cancer: surgical morbidity and intermediate follow-up. Am J Obstet Gynecol 2002;187:340-8.

[56] Possover M, Krause N, Plaul K, Kuhne-Heid R, Schneider A. Laparoscopic para-aortic and pelvic lymphadenectomy: experience with 150 patients and review of literature. Gynecol Oncol. 1998;78:19-28.

[57] Bouwman F, Smits A, Lopes A, Das N, Pollard A, Massuger L, et al. The impact of BMI on surgical complications and outcomes in endometrial cancer surgery-An institutional study and systematic review of the literature. Gynecol Oncol 2015;139:369-76.

[58] Singh S, Swarer K, Resnick K. Longer operative time is associated with increased postoperative complications in patients undergoing minimally-invasive surgery for endometrial cancer. Gynecol Oncol 2017;147:554-7.

[59] Jansen FW, Kolkman W, Bakkum EA, De Kroon CD, Trimbos-Kemper TCM, Trimbos JB. Complications of laparoscopy: an inquiry about closed- versus open-entry technique. Am J Obstet Gynecol 2004;190:634-8.

[60] Zikan M, Fischerova D, Pinkavova I, Slama J, Weinberger V, Dusek L, et al. A prospective study examining the incidence of asymptomatic and symptomatic lymphoceles following lymphadenectomy in patients with gynecological cancer. Gynecol Oncol 2015;137:291-8.

[61] Kohler C, Tozzi R, Klemm P, Schneider A. Laparoscopic paraaortic left-sided transperitoneal infraenal lymphadenectomy in patients with gynecologic malignancies: technique and results. Gynecol Oncol 2003;91:139-48.

[62] Bishop E, Java J, Moore K, Spirtos N, Pearl M, Zivanovitc O et al. Surgical outcomes among elderly women with endometrial cancer treated by laparoscopic hysterctomy: A NRG/ Gynecologic oncology Group Study. Am J Obstet Gynecol. 2018;218(1):109.e1- 109.e11.

[63] Kavoussi LR, Sosa E, Chandhoke P, Chodak G, Clayman RV, Hadley HR, et al. Complications of laparoscopic pelvic lymph node dissection. J Urol 1993;149:322-5.

[64] Freid RM, Siegel D, Smith AD, Weiss GH. Lymphoceles after laparoscopic pelvic node dissection. Urology 1998;51:131-4.

[65] Rahm C, Adok C, Dahm-Kahler P, Bohlin KS. Complications and risk factors in vulvar cancer surgery - A population-based study. Eur J Surg Oncol J Eur Soc Surg Oncol Br Assoc Surg Oncol 2022;48:1400-6.

[66] Touboul C, Uzan C, Mauguen A, Gouy S, Rey A, Pautier P, et al. Survival and prognostic factors after cloture surgery in patients with advanced stageë cervical cancer. Gynecologic' Obstëtrique Fertil 2011;39:274-80.

[67] Chemoradiotherapy for Cervical Cancer Meta-Analysis Collaboration. Reducing uncertainties about the effects of chemoradiotherapy for cervical cancer: a systematic review and meta-analysis of individual patient data from 18 randomized trials. J Clin Oncol Off J Am Soc Clin Oncol 2008;26:5802-12.

[68] Colombo N, Creutzberg C, Amant F, Bosse T, Gonzalez-Martin A, Ledermann J, et al. ESMO-ESGO-ESTRO Consensus Conference on Endometrial Cancer: Diagnosis, Treatment and Follow-up. Int J Gynecol Cancer Off J Int Gynecol Cancer Soc 2016;26:2-30.

7 APPENDICES

APPENDIX 1 :
ASA score (the American Society of anaesthesiologists)

SCORE ASA

Patient's state of health	Score
Patent sam, en borne santd, Cest a-dine sans attainte organique. physiologique. bichimique ou psychique	1
Malade syst6mique ldgdre, patient pr6$entant une attemte mod6r6e (Tune grande fonction, par example l6gdre hypertension, апбпие, bronchte chrorique ldgfcre	2
Severe or irreversible systemic disease. patent presenting a severe symptom of great severity which does not lead to incapacity, e.g. moderate heart failure. debate, severe hypertension, early cardiac decompensation.	3
Patent with severe impairment of a major function. disabling. and that the prognosis is vital, for example: chest engine at rest, pronounced systdmiquo rsuffisanco (pulmonary, rdnalc, hdpatic, cardiac ...].	4
Moribund patient whose life expectancy is less than 24 hours, with or without surgical intervention	5

APPENDIX 2:
FIGO 1988 ovarian cancer classification

UICC FIGO 1968		
T3 and/or N1	III	Tumour enlarging one or both ovaries with microscopically confirmed peritoneal metastasis(es) outside the pelvis and/or metastatic lymph node(s) found in both ovaries
T3a	II A	Microscopic metastases outside the pelvis
T3b	IIIB	Macroscopic peritoneal metastasis(es) outside the pelvis of 2 cm or less
T3c	me	Macroscopic peritoneal metastasis(es) outside the pelvis over 2 cm long and/or regional metastatic lymph node(s)

APPENDIX 3:
FIGO 1988 endometrial cancer classification

* Stage I :
- IA: non-invasive, limited to the endometrium
- IB: infiltration < 1/2 myometre thickness
- IC: infiltration " 1/2 myometre thickness

* Stage II:
- 11A: Microscopic invasion of endocervical glands
- HB: Invasion of cervical stroma

* Stage III:
- IIIA: serosal and/or adnexal involvement and/or positive peritoneal cytology
- IIIB: vaginal metastases
- IIIC: pelvic or paraaortic lymph node metastases

- Stage IV:
- VIA: mucosal involvement (> bullous oedema) of the bladder or rectum
- IVB: abdominal metastasis(es) and/or & distance and/or N+ inguinal

APPENDIX 4:

FIGO 2009 endometrial cancer classification

Nouvelle classification FIGO

FIGO (2009)[20]	TNM (2009)[22]	DESCRIPTION	FIGO (1989)
Stades I*	T1	Tumeur limitée au corps utérin	Stades I
IA	T1a	Tumeur limitée à l'endomètre ou ne dépassant pas la moitié du myomètre	IA-B
IB	T1b	Tumeur envahissant la moitié du myomètre ou plus de la moitié du myomètre	IC
Stades II*	T2	Tumeur envahissant le stroma cervical mais ne s'étendant pas au-delà de l'utérus	Stades IIA-B
Stades III*	T3 et/ou N1	Extensions locales et/ou régionales comme suit :	Stades III
IIIA	T3a	Séreuse et/ou annexes**	IIIA
IIIB	T3b	Envahissement vaginal et/ou paramétrial**	IIIB
IIIC	N1	Atteinte des ganglions lymphatiques régionaux**	IIIC
IIIC1		Ganglions pelviens	
IIIC2		Ganglions lomboaortiques +/- ganglions pelviens	
Stades IV*	T4 et/ou M1	Extension à la muqueuse vésicale et/ou intestinale et/ou métastases à distance	Stades IV
IVA	T4	Extension à la muqueuse vésicale et/ou intestinale	IVA
IVB	M1	Métastases à distance incluant les métastases intra-abdominales et/ou ganglions inguinaux	IVB

*: grades 1, 2 ou 3 ; **: Les résultats de la cytologie péritonéale doivent être rapportés séparément et ne modifient pas la classification (la classification FIGO de 1989 incluait les résultats d'une cytologie positive pour les stades IIIA).

Grades 1, 2 or 3 **: Results of peritoneal cytdogy must be reported separately and do not alter the classification (the 1989 FIGO classification included the results of positive cytology for stages IIIA).

APPENDIX 5:

FIGO ovarian cancer classification 2013 vs 1988

		Old-1988 FIGO stage			New - 2013 FIGO stage
Stage 1	IA	Tumor limited to one ovary, capsule intact, no tumor on ovarian surface, and negative washings/ascites	IA		Tumor limited to one ovary or fallopian tube, capsule intact, no tumor on surface, and negative washings/ascites
	IB	Tumor involves both ovaries, capsule intact, no tumor on ovarian surface, and negative washings/ascites	IB		Tumor limited to both ovaries or fallopian tubes, capsule intact, no tumor on surface, and negative washings/ascites
	IC	Tumor limited to ovaries with any of the following: capsule rupture, tumor on ovarian surface, or positive washing/ascites	IC		Tumor limited to one or both ovaries or fallopian tube
			IC1		- With surgical spill
			IC2		"With capsule rupture before surgery or tumor on ovarian or fallopian tube surface
			IC3		- With malignant cells in the ascites or peritoneal washings

APPENDIX 6:

FIGO endometrial cancer classification 2018

Stadium	Tumour confined to the uterine body
IA	Tumour confined to the endometrium or invading less than half the myometrium
IB	Tumour invading half or more of the myometrium
Stage IIB]	Tumour invading the cervical stroma but not beyond the uterus
	Local and/or regional extensions with the following characteristics:

Stage III™	
IDA	Tumour invasion of the serosa of the uterine body or adnexa (direct or metastatic extension)[131]
IIIB	Vaginal or parametrial invasion (direct or metastatic extension),[31]
IIIC	Involvement of pelvic or para-aortic lymph nodesd ⤶
IIIC1 IIIC2	Involvement of pelvic lymph nodes
Stage r	Para-aortic lymph node involvement with or without pelvic lymph node involvement
IVA	Extension to the vesicular and/or intestinal mucosa and/or distant metastases
	Extension to the vesicular and/or intestinal mucosa
IVB	Metastases ŭ distance including intra-abdominal metastases eVor inguinal lymph nodes excluding vaginal, adnexal or pelvic serous metastases

1. t^1 Grades 1, 2 or 3

2. t^2 Endocen/icai glandular invasion should be considered as a siade I

3. T^3 Pentontal cytology results may be reported separately and do not affect the classification.

4. Bullous oedema on cystoscopy is insufficient to be considered stage IV (NCCN, 2019).

<u>APPENDIX 7:</u>
FIGO Ovarian Cancer Classification 2018

T	N	M	Stades FIGO	Définition
T1	N0	M0	Stade I	Tumeur limitée aux ovaires (1 ou les 2)
T1a	N0	M0	Stade IA	Tumeur limitée à un seul ovaire ; capsule intacte, sans tumeur à la surface de l'ovaire ; pas de cellule maligne dans le liquide d'ascite ou de lavage péritonéal
T1b	N0	M0	Stade IB	Tumeur limitée aux deux ovaires ; capsules intactes, sans tumeur à la surface de l'ovaire ; pas de cellule maligne dans le liquide d'ascite ou de lavage péritonéal
T1c	N0	M0	Stade IC *	Tumeur limitée à 1 ou aux 2 ovaires, avec : • soit rupture capsulaire • soit tumeur à la surface des ovaires • soit cellules malignes présentes dans le liquide d'ascite ou de lavage péritonéal
T2	N0	M0	Stade II	Tumeur intéressant 1 ou les 2 ovaires avec extension pelvienne
T2a	N0	M0	Stade IIA	Extension et/ou greffes utérines et/ou tubaires ; pas de cellule maligne dans le liquide d'ascite ou le liquide de lavage péritonéal
T2b	N0	M0	Stade IIB	Extension à d'autres organes pelviens ; pas de cellule maligne dans le liquide d'ascite ou le liquide de lavage péritonéal
T3	et/ou N1	M0	Stade III	Tumeur de l'ovaire avec extension péritonéale abdominale et/ou ganglionnaire rétropéritonéale
T3a	N0	M0	Stade IIIA **	Métastases rétropéritonéales microscopiques ± péritoine
T3b	N0	M0	Stade IIIB	Métastases péritonéales extra-pelviennes ≤ 2 cm ± adénopathies
T3c	et/ou N1	M0	Stade IIIC	Métastases péritonéales extra-pelviennes >2 cm ± adénopathies
Tous T	Tous N	M1	Stade IV ***	Métastases à distance (à l'exclusion des métastases péritonéales)

- * : stade IC
  - IC1 : rupture peropératoire
  - IC2 : rupture préopératoire ou végétations en surface
  - IC3 : cellules malignes dans l'ascite ou le liquide de lavage péritonéal
- ** : stade IIIA
  - IIIA1 : adénopathie rétropéritonéale seule (prouvé par cytologie histologie)
    - IIIA1(i) : foyer adénocarcinomateux dans l'adénopathie ≤ 10 mm
    - IIIA1(ii) : foyer adénocarcinomateux dans l'adénopathie >10 mm
  - IIIA2 : extension péritonéale microscopique extrapelvienne ± adénopathies
- *** : stade IV : cancer de l'ovaire avec métastases à distance
  - IVA : plèvre (cytologie positive)
  - IVB : autres métastases y compris adénopathies inguinales

APPENDIX 8:
FIGO Cervical Cancer Classification 2018

4.1. Stade I

- La classification FIGO peut maintenant être basée sur l'examen clinique, l'imagerie ou l'anatomo-pathologie selon le bilan effectué ; l'atteinte ganglionnaire est à préciser à part

Cancer strictement limité au col		
Stade IA	Cancer invasif identifié seulement au microscope et envahissement du stroma : profondeur maximum de 5 mm	
	IA1	profondeur $\leq$ 3 mm, largeur $\leq$ 7 mm
	IA2	3 mm < profondeur $\leq$ 5 mm et largeur $\leq$ 7 mm
Stade IB	Cancer clinique limité au col visible en macroscopie ou cancer microscopique de dimension supérieure au IA	
	IB1	T <2 cm
	IB2	2 $\leq$ T <4 cm
	IB3	T $\geq$ 4 cm

4.2. Stade II

Cancer étendu au-delà du col mais n'atteignant pas la paroi pelvienne ni le tiers inférieur du vagin		
Stade IIA	jusqu'aux deux tiers supérieurs du vagin	
	IIA1	Taille T $\leq$ 4 cm
	IIA2	Taille T >4 cm
Stade IIB	paramètres (proximaux)	

Remarque : une conisation à marge+ est à considérer comme IB1 (Bhatla, 2018)

4.3. Stade III

Cancer étendu jusqu'à la paroi pelvienne et/ou au tiers inférieur du vagin (y compris hydronéphrose)		
Stade IIIA		Atteinte vaginale jusqu'au tiers inférieur
Stade IIIB		Fixation à la paroi pelvienne (ou hydronéphrose ou rein muet)
Stade IIIC	IIIC1	Atteinte ganglionnaire pelvienne *
	IIIC2	Atteinte ganglionnaire lombo-aortique *

* Préciser si atteinte sur imagerie (IIIC1r ou IIIC2r) ou sur l'anatomo-pathologie (IIIC1p ou IIIC2p)

- En cas de curage ganglionnaire, la présence de cellules isolées (<0.2 mm) ou de micrométastases (0,2 à 2,0 mm) ne change pas la classification car leur implication pronostique n'est pas claire ; leur présence doit être notée dans le dossier.

4.4. Stade IV

Cancer étendu au-delà du petit bassin ou à la muqueuse vésicale et/ou rectale	
Stade IVA	Organe adjacent (vessie, rectum)
Stade IVB	A distance

APPENDIX 9:
Histological classification of endometrial cancer according to WHO

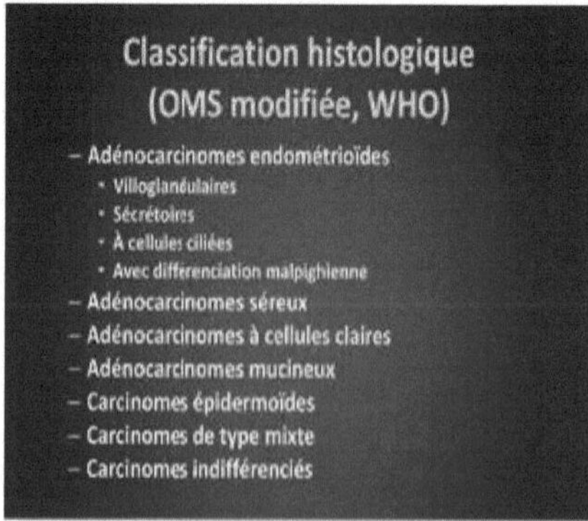

Histological classification of ovarian cancer according to WHO and FIGO

Classification (OMS et FIGO)

A/ Tumeurs épithéliales communes(Les + fréquentes : 80%)

B/ Tumeurs des cellules germinales (env. 10%)

C/ Tumeurs endocrines (3,7%)

D/ Tumeurs conjonctives

D/ Tumeurs métastatiques

E/ Tumeurs de l'ovaire non spécifiques

APPENDIX 11 :

Histological classification of cervical cancer according to WHO

Tumeurs épithéliales

Tumeurs épidermoïdes et précurseurs

Carcinome épidermoïde (SAI)

Kératinisant

Non kératinisant

A cellules basales

Verruqueux

Condylomateux

Papillaire

Lymphoépithélial

A cellules transitionnelles

Carcinome épidermoïde avec invasion précoce (micro invasif)

Néoplasie intraépithéliale épidermoïde

Néoplasie cervicale intraépithéliale (CIN3)

Carcinome épidermoïde in situ

Lésions cellulaires épidermoïdes bénignes

Condylome accuminé

APPENDIX 12 :
Classintra 2020 classification of intraoperative complications

Grade	Definition	Examples
Grade 0	No deviation from the ideal intraoperative course	
Grade I	Any deviation from the ideal intraoperative course • Without the need for any additional treatment or intervention • Patient asymptomatic or mild symptoms	• **Bleeding:** Bleeding above average from small-calibre vessel; self-limiting or definitively manageable without additional treatment than routine coagulation • **Injury:** Minimal serosal intestinal lesion, not requiring any additional treatment • **Cautery:** Small burn of the skin, no treatment necessary • **Arrhythmia:** arrhythmia (e.g. extrasystoles) without relevance
Grade II	Any deviation from the ideal intraoperative course • With the need for any additional minor treatment or intervention • Patient with moderate symptoms, not life-threatening; and not leading to permanent disability	• **Bleeding:** Bleeding from medium calibre artery or vein, ligation, use of tranexamic acid • **Injury:** Non-transmural intestinal lesion requiring suture(s) • **Cautery:** Moderate burn requiring non-invasive wound care • **Arrhythmia:** Arrhythmia requiring administration of antiarrhythmic drug, no hemodynamic effect
Grade III	Any deviation from the ideal intraoperative course • With the need for any additional moderate treatment or intervention • Patient with severe symptoms, potentially life-threatening, and/or potentially leading to permanent disability	• **Bleeding:** Bleeding from large calibre artery or vein with transient hemodynamic instability, ligation or suture; blood transfusion • **Injury:** Transmural intestinal lesion requiring segmental resection • **Cautery:** Severe burn requiring surgical debridement • **Arrhythmia:** Arrhythmia requiring administration of antiarrhythmic drug, transient hemodynamic effect
Grade IV	Any deviation from the ideal intraoperative course • With the need for any additional major and urgent treatment or intervention • Patient with life-threatening symptoms and/or leading to permanent disability	• **Bleeding:** Life-threatening bleeding with splenectomy, massive blood transfusion, ICU stay • **Injury:** Injury of central artery or vein requiring extended intestinal resection • **Cautery:** Life-threatening burn injury by cautery leading to fire requiring ICU treatment • **Arrhythmia:** Arrhythmia requiring electroconversion, defibrillator or admission to the ICU
Grade V	Any deviation from the ideal intraoperative course • With intraoperative death of the patient	

The following events are not defined as intraoperative adverse events: sequelae, failures of cure, events not related to the underlying disease, wrong-site or wrong-patient surgery or errors in indication.

Grade I	Tout évènement post-opératoire indésirable ne nécessitant pas de traitement médical, chirurgical, endoscopique ou radiologique. Les seuls traitements autorisés sont les antiémétiques, antipyrétiques, antalgiques, diurétiques, électrolytes et la physiothérapie.	Iléus, abcès de paroi mis à plat au chevet du patient
Grade II	Complication nécessitant un traitement médical n'étant pas autorisé dans le grade 1.	Thrombose veineuse périphérique, nutrition parentérale totale, transfusion
Grade III	Complication nécessitant un traitement chirurgical, endoscopique ou radiologique.	
IIIa	Sans anesthésie générale	Ponction guidée radiologiquement
IIIb	Sous anesthésie générale	Reprise chirurgicale pour saignement ou autre cause
Grade IV	Complication engageant le pronostic vital et nécessitant des soins intensifs	
IVa	Défaillance d'un organe	Dialyse
IVb	Défaillance multi-viscérale	
Grade V	Décès	

Resume

Problem: The place of lumbo-aortic curage remains a controversial subject in the literature, given the difficulty of carrying it out and the non-negligible number of intra- and post-operative complications. Identification of the factors limiting lumbo-aortic curage and the intra- and post-operative complications, on the one hand, and study of its impact on the carcinological prognosis of patients, on the other hand, remain essential in deciding on its indication.

Aims of the work :

- To clarify the indications and limitations of lumbo-aortic curage.
- To describe the intra- and post-operative complications of lumbo-aortic curage.
- To study the impact of curage on the prognosis of patients with pelvic gynecological cancer.
- Based on our series and a recent review of the literature, to determine the current role of lumbo-aortic curage in the treatment of gynaecological cancers.

Materials and methods: We carried out a single-centre, retrospective, descriptive, analytical and comparative study of 85 patients operated on for gynaecological cancer with an indication for lumboaortic curage, over a 19-year period from January 2003 to December 2021, in the obstetric gynaecology department of the Ben Arous regional hospital.

Results: The following factors were statistically correlated with failure to perform lumbo-aortic curage: body mass index ($p=0.02$) and obesity in particular ($p=0.033$), the presence of complications during pelvic curage ($p=0.002$), the type of cancer ($p=0.05$) and the years of experience of the surgical team ($p=0.04$). In total, we noted the presence of 30 intraoperative complications: Grade 1: 15 (50%), Grade 2: 8 (26.7%), Grade 3: 6 (20%), Grade 4: 1 (3.3%).

In a multivariate study, lumbo-aortic curage appeared to significantly increase the 3-year recurrence-free survival rate ($p=0.02$), irrespective of the patient's age, the stage of the disease and the time between diagnosis and the start of treatment.

Conclusion: The major factors limiting lumbo-aortic curage are the occurrence of per-operative complications during pelvic curage and the experience of the surgeon. However, when it is performed, lumbo-aortic curage does not carry a significantly greater risk of complications than isolated pelvic curage, and it increases overall survival and recurrence-free survival at 3 years.

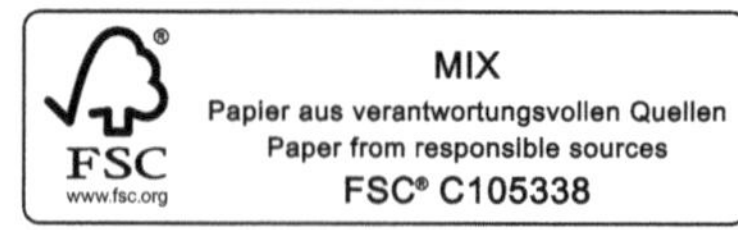

Printed by Books on Demand GmbH, Norderstedt / Germany